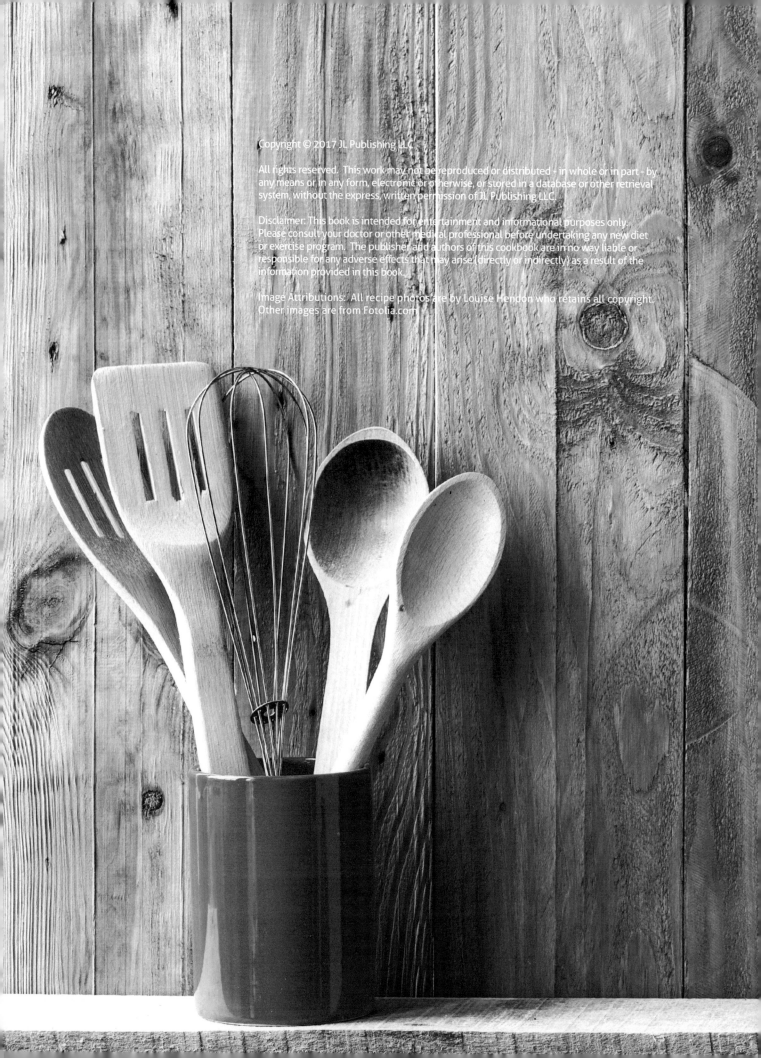

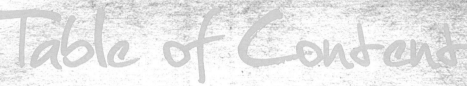
Table of Contents

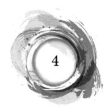

Food as Medicine & Cooking for Life

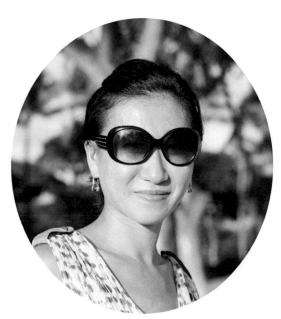

I have an autoimmune disease. And for a long time, I felt like I was the only one.

But in truth, there are at least 50 million other Americans with an autoimmune disease. That's a LOT.

I'm sure that your experience is different than mine. But I also suspect that you might sometimes feel the same way as I have...

Frustrated and Helpless, Like the Medical System is Failing You

Modern medicine is amazing in so many ways. For instance, infant mortality is lower than ever. And you could break twenty bones and be fully recovered a year from now.

But modern medicine is not great at curing chronic illnesses like autoimmune diseases. And that's frustrating.

I visited doctor after doctor for many years, and they ran more tests than I can remember. But nobody ever offered me a real solution to my illness.

At best, they prescribed me medication to treat and mask my symptoms.

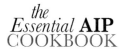
the
Essential **AIP**
COOKBOOK

I don't blame any of those doctors. They didn't know what to do.

But I was constantly disappointed. And I've talked to a lot of people who feel the exact same way.

Fortunately, I found a way to heal my body without medication…

Real Food is the Key to Real Health

For as long as I can remember, I have loved eating.

And for most of my life, I loved eating junk food. After all, junk food is chemically designed to be addictive.

But once I started struggling to heal my body, something had to change. It was my change to Paleo and Real Food that made more difference than anything else.

I hated being sick, but there was a silver lining…

Once I understood the impact of food on my body, I also learned to appreciate and love whole, fresh foods. Today, I eat better than ever, in terms of both health AND taste.

Better yet, I look forward to cooking, which was never the case when I was younger. Until recently, I viewed cooking as a chore that would take up what little time I had.

Today, I view it as a fun and exciting opportunity to create delicious food and make myself feel better.

And that's what I want to share with you and with the world…

A Love for Cooking, with a Little Perspective

I hated cooking for most of my life.

And for many years, I worked long hours as a lawyer in New York City. As you can guess, I had little desire or time to cook after getting home from a long day at the office.

So I understand completely that you may not look forward to cooking every day.

And yet, I believe that everybody can learn to enjoy cooking. I believe that cooking can bring friends and family together like few other activities. And cooking does not need to be complicated or time-consuming.

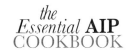

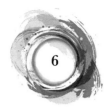

Most of all, if you have an autoimmune disease, cooking is one of the most powerful things you can do to heal your body.

That's why I wrote this cookbook for a Paleo Autoimmune Protocol.

Healing Your Body
Can Be Fun and Easy

Healing your body is not easy every single day. But it doesn't need to be a lifelong struggle. Getting well can also be much more fun than you think.

And getting better definitely starts in the kitchen. There are some amazing restaurants and great health-food brands. Still, 99% of restaurants and prepared foods are suspect at best.

If you're trying to heal an autoimmune disease, then almost all the food you eat needs to be cooked at home.

But that's hard if each meal takes you hours to prepare.

I Believe in Simple, Fast, & Easy Recipes

It sounds silly, but I think most recipes should be simple, fast, & easy. On special occasions, I sometimes choose to make complex and time-consuming dishes.

On normal days, I don't have the time or energy to cook all day.

With just a couple exceptions, all recipes in this book are easy and quick to make. Plus, they turn out well each and every time.

Because if any one of those things isn't true, then cooking becomes much less fun.

When that happens, you're likely to revert back to eating foods that don't heal or nourish your body.

Let's Build a Better Life

This is just a cookbook.

But I also view it as much more than that.

I view this as an opportunity for you to dramatically improve your health and your life. A chance to take control of your body and feel younger, healthier, and happier.

Most of all, I view it as a tool for you to live a life that you love.

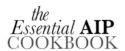

A 4-Step Guide To Healing Autoimmune Diseases

This is a cookbook, so you'll find a lot of great recipes that follow the autoimmune protocol diet (AIP).

But I know first-hand that healing an autoimmune disease is tough. If you're just getting started on your journey of healing, then you need a plan.

So besides recipes, I've also included below my 4-Step Guide to Healing an Autoimmune Disease.

This is more of a general template than an exact plan. Your experience will be different than anybody else's experience. But this guide will hopefully help you get started in the best way possible.

First of all, we need to start here...

What is an Autoimmune Disease?

When the doctor first told me I had an autoimmune disease, I had no clue what he was talking about, so in case you're also confused, let's start with what an autoimmune disease is.

An autoimmune disease is when your body's immune system attacks other parts of your body. Normally, your immune system would attack only 'foreign' invaders like germs.

The consequences of an autoimmune disease depend on the particular disease that you have. But these diseases often result in widespread destruction of organs and cells.

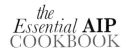

Here are a few Common Autoimmune Diseases:

- *Hashimoto's Thyroiditis*
- *Graves' Disease*
- *Type 1 Diabetes*
- *Rheumatoid Arthritis*
- *Psoriasis*
- *Celiac Disease*
- *Crohn's Disease*

- *Lupus*
- *Narcolepsy*
- *Ulcerative Colitis*
- *Multiple Sclerosis*
- *Guillain-Barré Syndrome*
- *Hidradenitis Suppurativa*
- *Alopecia Areata*
- *Autoimmune Hepatitis*
- *Angioedema (the disease that I have)*

Why Food is So Important for Healing

You might already know that food is important in healing your autoimmune disease. It's important that you know exactly why.

If you know why food is so important, you're more likely to stick to a healing AIP diet. And you're also better able to make changes when you need to.

The primary job of your intestines is to let some stuff through (into your bloodstream) and to keep out other stuff.

In general, your intestines will absorb digested food and allow it into your bloodstream. That way, your body is able to get nutrition from digested food.

Your intestines will keep almost everything else out of your bloodstream. That includes undigested food, bacteria, etc.

Unfortunately, your intestines can stop working properly sometimes. When that happens, the result is often that too many things are allowed to pass into your bloodstream. That's not a good thing. You don't want bacteria, viruses, or undigested food in your bloodstream.

Your body does have a second line of defense. When bacteria and other pathogens pass into your bloodstream, your immune system attacks them.

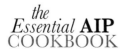

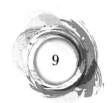

It's good that your immune system attacks 'foreign' objects in your bloodstream. That's how you fight off illness and infection.

But there's also a downside. If a lot of things are making it into your blood, your immune system will sometimes make mistakes.

One big mistake is that it will start to attack parts of your own body. To your immune system, 'foreign' objects (like undigested food) can sometimes resemble parts of your body.

And that's one of the primary ways that an autoimmune disease occurs.

The food you eat is very important in two ways. First of all, food is often the cause of your intestines not working properly. It's not the only cause, but it's a big one.

Moreover, food is what will allow your intestines to heal or else stay broken. And healing your intestines is critical for healing your autoimmune disease.

What is the Paleo Autoimmune Protocol (AIP)?

The Autoimmune Protocol was developed by Dr. Loren Cordain and Robb Wolf (see the "Autoimmune Caveat" in Robb Wolf's The Paleo Solution).

It's a variation of a Paleo diet to help those with autoimmune diseases. In particular, you must remove certain foods for a time. Later, you can reintroduce those foods to see how your body reacts.

In the Appendix at the end of this book, I've included a detailed AIP food list. This list shows both foods that you can eat and also foods to avoid. I've also included a basic AIP food list in the next chapter to give you an overview.

Sarah Ballantyne has written more about healing autoimmune

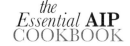

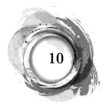

conditions in her book, The Paleo Approach. And check out the resources listed at the end of this book if you wish to do further reading on autoimmune conditions.

The basic idea behind the autoimmune protocol is to remove problem foods for at least 60 days to allow your body to heal. That also allows you to set a baseline of how good you can feel.

By doing this, you can discover how your body reacts to various foods. You can also begin healing your body.

Who Should Try a Paleo Autoimmune Protocol?

The Paleo Autoimmune Protocol is not easy. It requires some hard work.

But if you have an autoimmune disease, then this is your diet. Healing your autoimmune disease can change your life. And to do that, you must remove the foods that are making you sick.

You have everything to gain and little to lose.

But it requires a commitment. Trying it for just 4-5 days is NOT going to help. It takes time and dedication to heal your body.

With that in mind, here is how I suggest getting started.

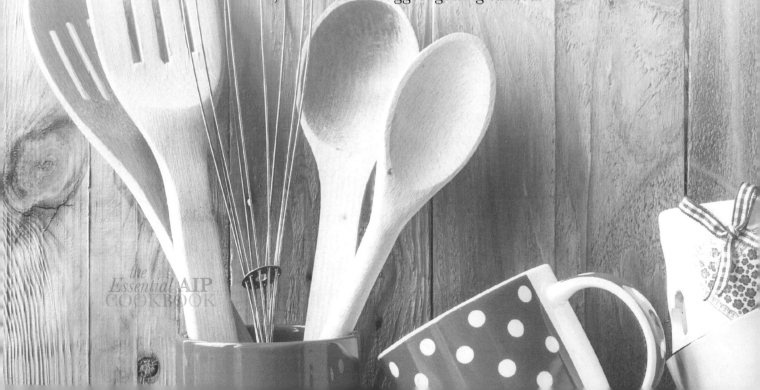

4 Steps to Healing
Autoimmune Diseases:

1. Make a Commitment.

It sounds obvious, but you need to admit that it's going to be a bit of a lifestyle change for the next few months (at least). Tell your friends and family what you're doing and why, so that they'll help and support you.

2. 60 Days of Elimination.

This is where this cookbook comes in. For 60 days, you need to remove all foods that may be causing you problems. (See the next chapter for what foods to eliminate.) All recipes in this cookbook contain only foods that you can eat during this elimination period.

Of course, if you have sensitivities to foods that are generally considered OK on an autoimmune protocol, then you should eliminate those foods too.

3. Start Re-Introducing One Food at a Time.

After 60 days, continue to cook meals with no problematic ingredients. However, also start introducing one ingredient for a few days at a time.

4. Record How You Feel, then Rinse and Repeat.

Keep a list of foods that make you feel worse when you reintroduce them. Also keep a list of foods that don't make you feel worse. Then keep going through ingredients until you know exactly which foods cause you trouble. If you need to, repeat steps 1-4 every year or so, as the results will often change over time.

Optional Step #5: TEST.

This is not a required step. Many people have healed their bodies without testing. But if you can afford it, testing can help you heal much faster.

When you have an autoimmune condition, a few things happen. First, your body often depletes many of the nutrients you need to be healthy. Second, your body becomes a great host for pathogens like parasites and bacteria. Third, many processes in your body stop working as well.

The good news is that almost everything is reversible.

But if you don't address specific problems, then healing can take longer. For instance, if you have a parasite in your gut, then it may take years to heal, rather than just months.

That's why I highly encourage testing if you can afford it. In particular, work with someone who will run the following tests:

• Urine Organic Acids (preferably from Genova Labs).
• Comprehensive Stool Analysis (preferably from Biohealth Labs).
• NutrEval (Genova Labs) or Spectracell Micronutrient Profile.
• Adrenal Stress Profile (preferably from Biohealth Labs).

Most doctors are not familiar with these tests and will not run them. And most insurance will not cover the costs.

But these tests will uncover almost any underlying issues that may keep you from getting healthy.

As I mentioned, you can follow the 4-step approach above and get amazing results. This is an optional step. But it's one that I recommend if you can do it.

If you're looking for someone to run these tests, please check out http://nourishbalancethrive.com.

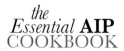

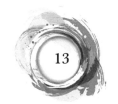

Common Mistakes on AIP

Finally, I also want to alert you to 2 common mistakes that people make on a Paleo Autoimmune Protocol:

Mistake #1: Only Changing Your Diet And Nothing Else.

Stress, lack of sleep, and lack of exercise are huge components of AIP that many people miss. Change your diet, but please don't overlook these other factors.

Mistake #2: Eating Foods that You're Sensitive To.

Even if a certain food is allowed on AIP, you might still be sensitive to it (e.g., coconut products). If you suspect a food might be causing a problem for you, then treat it as a "not allowed" food. You can always reintroduce it after the elimination period.

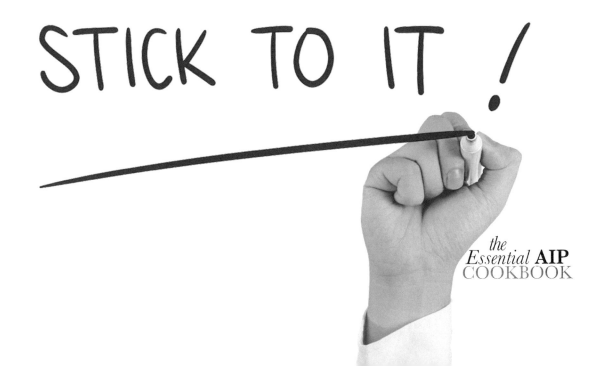

STICK TO IT !

the
Essential **AIP**
COOKBOOK

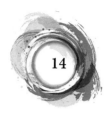

Basic AIP Food List

A very detailed list is attached at the end of this book (you can also get a printable PDF version here: http://paleomagazine.com/aip-food-list), but here are some categories of foods to watch out for (of course, all the recipes in this cookbook are complaint with the autoimmune protocol and do not contain any of the foods on the not allowed list):

FOODS NOT ALLOWED ON BASIC PALEO DIET
No Grains (including rice and quinoa)
No Dairy
No Legumes (including soy and peanuts)
No Sugars
No Vegetable or Seed Oils
No Additives (typically fine if you avoid all processed foods)

ADDITIONAL FOODS NOT ALLOWED ON AIP
No Eggs (including even paleo mayo)
No Nuts
No Seeds (including cocoa*, coffee*, seed-based spices*)
No Nightshades (including, tomatoes, eggplants/aubergines, potatoes, peppers, and any pepper-based spices - see the detailed list in Appendix A)
No Alcohol*
No NSAIDS* (including aspirin, ibuprofen)
No Stevia*
No Emulsifiers* or thickeners (e.g., guar gum, carrageenan)
Limit fruit to 2-5 servings per day*
No Algae* (including chlorella and spirulina)

FOODS YOU SHOULD EAT ON AIP
Vegetables (but avoid any nightshades, and note that corn, wheat, and rice are not vegetables)
Fruits (Sarah Ballantyne recommends limiting to 2-5 servings per day)

Meats, in particular organ meats
Bone broth is especially encouraged by many people
Seafood
Healthy fats
Fermented foods
Herbs (see more detailed list in Appendix A)

* indicates an additional limitation in stricter versions of the AIP diet (like that recommended by Sarah Ballantyne in The Paleo Approach)

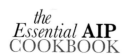

IN STRICTER VERSIONS OF AIP, TAKE SPECIAL CARE WITH
AVOIDING THE FOLLOWING FOODS AS THEY OFTEN CAUSE
CONFUSION FOR PEOPLE:

nutmeg	goji berries	cardamom
cacao	black pepper	coconut sugar
vanilla	allspice	stevia
coffee	star anise	ghee

Key AIP Pantry Ingredients

While no specific food is essential for an AIP diet, the following ingredients
will help to make your AIP diet more enjoyable and flavorful if you can
get a hold of them. By, the way, if you need help meal planning, then I've
included a 4-week AIP meal plan at the back of this book, and you can
download another one (that includes just slow cooker recipes or fast easy
dinner recipes) here: http://paleomagazine.com/aip-meal-plan

COCONUT AMINOS
This is a great non-soy alternative to soy sauce.

FISH SAUCE
A naturally AIP flavor-enhancing sauce. Make sure to get pure fish sauce.

COCONUT FLOUR
Great for creating a "bread-like" coating on fish and meats.

GARLIC POWDER
Adds a ton of flavor on meats.

ITALIAN SEASONING
An easy combination of AIP herbs. Make sure no non-AIP spices are
included in any seasoning mixes you purchase. (Some Italian seasoning
contain black or red pepper.)

ARROWROOT FLOUR/POWDER
Derived from a tropical plant, this is great for making AIP baked goods or for thickening your soups and sauces.

COCONUT MILK/CREAM
A non-dairy alternative for adding creaminess to recipes. Look for brands without thickeners like guar gum (as those ingredients are not AIP-friendly).

CAROB POWDER
This is great as an alternative to cacao.

GELATIN POWDER
Adding gelatin powder to your recipes is an excellent way to get more gelatin into your diet and it can act as a binder in many recipes.

CINNAMON POWDER
Perfect for adding extra flavor to desserts.

BONE BROTH (See Page 183 for recipe)
Great as a quick snack or for making soups. Make large batches of bone broth and freeze to use when necessary. Or keep a slow cooker going with bone broth so you can have it available any time.

OLIVE OIL
A good olive oil can add a ton of flavor to salads.

AVOCADO OIL/COCO OIL
These are versatile and healthy oils that are great for cooking with.

RAW HONEY
A good local raw honey can add hints of flowers and local plants that will amaze your senses.

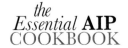

Chapter 1: Breakfast

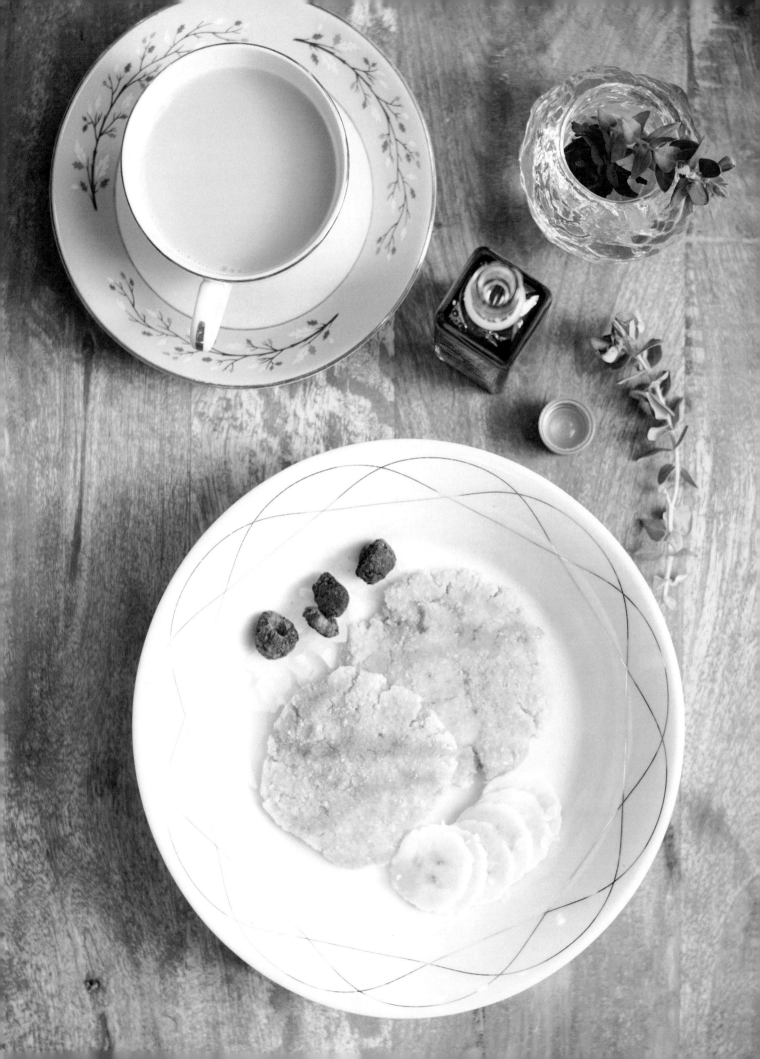

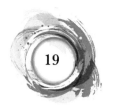

Amazing Banana Pancakes

Prep Time: 10 minutes
Cook Time: 20 minutes
Total Time: 30 minutes
Yield: 2 servings
Serving Size: 2 pancakes

These pancakes are amazing - they are soft but won't fall apart when cooked right.

I've found that these pancakes are best made in the oven. If you want to try making them in the frying pan with some coconut oil, then they will still taste great, but they do fall apart really easily so be very careful. Also don't let the pancakes cool too much because the gelatin in the mixture will make them chewy.

INGREDIENTS
- 1/2 bananas mashed
- 1/4 cup *(28 g)* coconut flour
- 1/8 teaspoon *(0.5 g)* baking soda
- 1 Tablespoon *(15 ml)* coconut oil
- 1 Tablespoon *(15 ml)* raw honey or maple syrup
- 1 Tablespoon *(7 g)* gelatin
- 3 Tablespoons *(45 ml)* hot water
- Extra raw honey or maple syrup *(for serving)*

INSTRUCTIONS
1. Preheat oven to 300 F *(150 C)*.
2. Place the mashed bananas, coconut flour, baking soda, coconut oil, and honey/maple syrup into a mixing bowl. Dissolve the gelatin in the hot water and then add into the mixing bowl as well.
3. Mix well to form batter.
4. Make the batter into around a golf-ball size and press down to a pancake of around 1/4-inch *(0.6 cm)* thick. Batter should make 4 pancakes.
5. Bake for 20 minutes and remove carefully from oven. Cool a little and then eat. Drizzle with extra honey or maple syrup if desired.

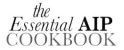

the Essential **AIP** COOKBOOK

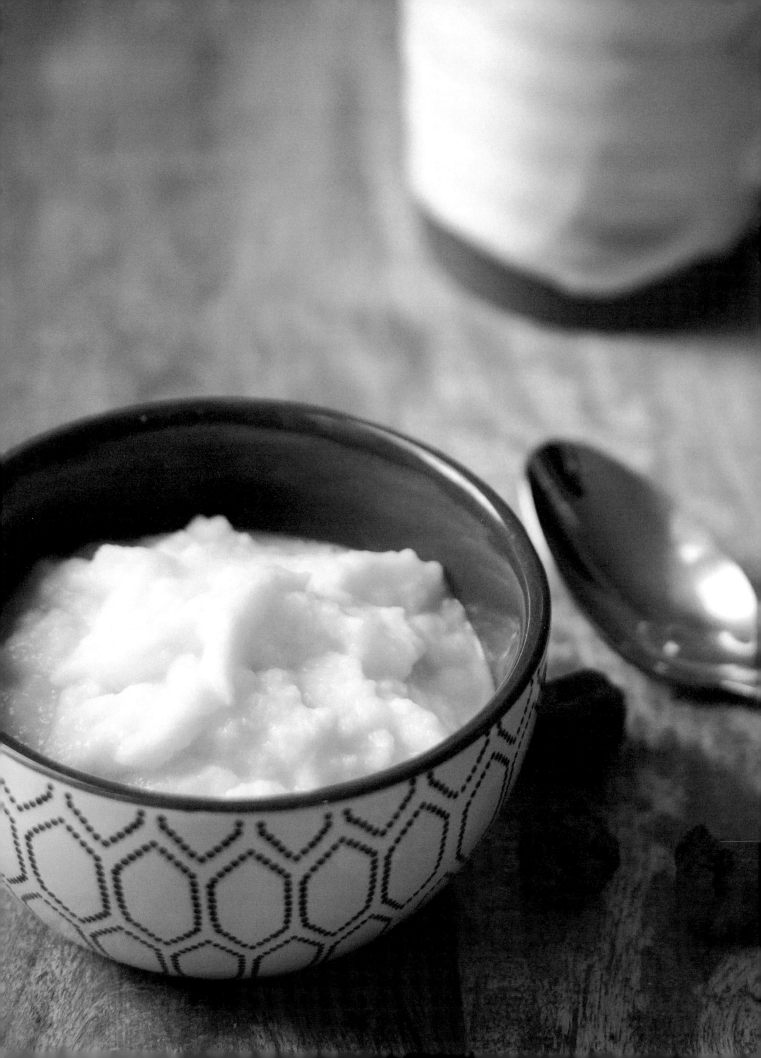

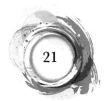

Apple Cauliflower Porridge

Prep Time: 10 minutes
Cook Time: 0 minutes
Total Time: 10 minutes
Yield: 2 servings
Serving Size: 1 bowl

Cauliflower is an amazing substitute for a lot of foods - in this recipe, the cauliflower provides a soft and creamy texture and the apple provides the sweetness that makes this breakfast recipe a sure winner.

Make sure to buy coconut milk without thickeners like guar gum.

INGREDIENTS
- 1 apple, peeled and chopped into large chunks
- 1/2 cauliflower *(approx. 10 oz or 280 g)* broken into florets and softened in microwave or steamed
- Dash of cinnamon
- 1/2 cup *(120 ml)* coconut milk or water

INSTRUCTIONS
1. Steam the cauliflower florets (or microwave it with some water in a bowl) to soften it.
2. Place the apple, cauliflower, cinnamon, and coconut milk/water into a blender.
3. Blend well and serve.

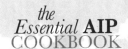
the **AIP**
Essential **AIP**
COOKBOOK

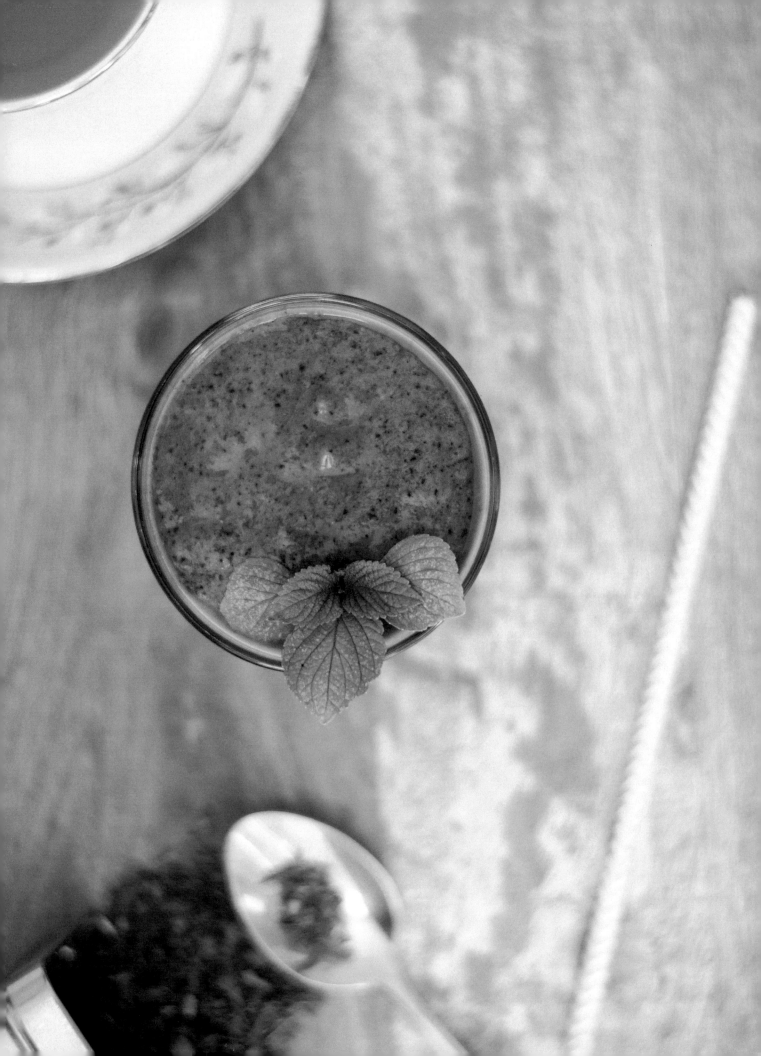

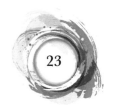

Blueberry Mint Smoothie

Prep Time: 5 minutes
Cook Time: 0 minutes
Total Time: 5 minutes
Yield: 1 serving
Serving Size: 1 glass

I love how refreshing the mint leaves make the smoothie. And the coconut milk and avocado create a delicious creamy texture.

INGREDIENTS

- 1/2 cup *(95 g)* frozen blueberries
- 1/2 cup *(120 ml)* coconut milk *(or water)*
- 1 teaspoon mint tea leaves *(or use approx. 10 fresh mint leaves)*
- 1/2 avocado
- 3/4 cup *(180 ml)* of ice

INSTRUCTIONS

1. Add everything to the blender.
2. Blend well.

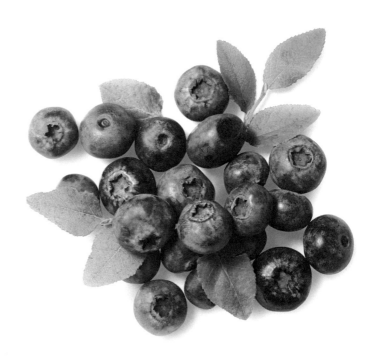

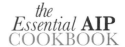

Bone Broth Noodle Soup

Prep Time: 5 minutes
Cook Time: 5 minutes
Total Time: 10 minutes
Yield: 2 servings
Serving Size: 1 bowl

When I was visiting Vietnam, I was shocked to learn that pho *(made traditionally with bone broth)* was eaten often as a breakfast dish. And so I thought, well, why not drink a super nutritious broth for breakfast! You can skip adding anything into it and just drink the bone broth straight if you prefer.

INGREDIENTS
- 4 cups *(1 l)* of bone broth *(See recipe on Page 183)*
- 1 zucchini, shredded
- 1 lime, juiced
- 1/2 teaspoon *(0.8 g)* ginger, grated
- 1/2 teaspoon *(1 g)* cinnamon
- 10 basil leaves
- 1 Tablespoon *(2 g)* cilantro, chopped
- Salt *(to taste)*

INSTRUCTIONS
1. Bring the bone broth to a boil.
2. Add in the lime juice, grated ginger, cinnamon, and then the zucchini.
3. Boil for 2 minutes.
4. Add in the basil and cilantro and serve.

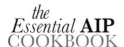

the
Essential AIP
COOKBOOK

Carrot and Apple Hash
with Cinnamon and Ginger

Prep Time: 10 minutes
Cook Time: 10 minutes
Total Time: 20 minutes
Yield: 2 servings
Serving Size: 1 small plate

When you taste this dish, you'll understand why it doesn't need any additional ingredients. The apple and carrots soften, and their natural sugars ooze out to mingle with the coconut oil making you savor every single bite of this dish. Perfect as a tasty side dish, snack, or for breakfast!

INGREDIENTS

- 1 medium carrot, shredded
- 1 apple, peeled and shredded
- 3 Tablespoons *(45 ml)* coconut oil *(for cooking)*
- Cinnamon *(for sprinkling)*
- Fresh ginger *(for topping)*

INSTRUCTIONS

1. Squeeze out any excess water from the shredded carrots and apples.
2. Mix the apples and carrots together and pour approx. 3 Tablespoons *(45 ml)* of coconut oil into the skillet/frying-pan.
3. Form the apple and carrot mixture into 2 large flat patties in the skillet/frying-pan and fry on medium heat *(2-3 minutes on each side – be careful when turning and check it doesn't burn).* Use a spatula to press down on the patties to help them cook better.
4. Serve with a sprinkling of cinnamon and freshly grated ginger.

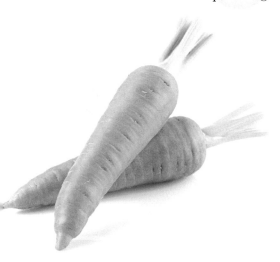

Carrot Apple Banana Smoothie

Prep Time: 5 minutes
Cook Time: 0 minutes
Total Time: 5 minutes
Yield: 1 serving
Serving Size: 1 glass

This is such an easy and delicious breakfast smoothie recipe. In fact, it's so delicious, you might find yourself wanting it for dessert too.

INGREDIENTS

- 1 apple, chopped
- 1/2 carrot *(approx. 3 oz or 85 g)*, chopped
- 1 banana
- 1 cup *(240 ml)* ice
- 1/2 Tablespoon *(7 ml)* coconut oil
- 1/2 cup *(120 ml)* coconut milk

INSTRUCTIONS

1. Place all the ingredients into a blender and blend well.

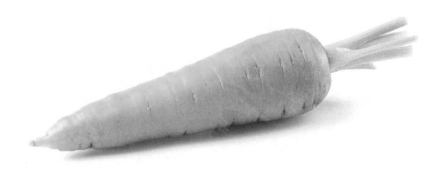

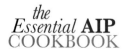

Chicken and Apple Sausages

Prep Time: 10 minutes
Cook Time: 20 minutes
Total Time: 30 minutes
Yield: 4 servings
Serving Size: 3 sausages

These can also be made in the oven if you prefer. I suggest making a large batch and then freezing the leftovers so you can reheat them for quick breakfasts in the morning.

INGREDIENTS

- 2 large chicken breasts, or use 1 lb *(454 g)* ground chicken
- 1 apple, peeled and finely diced
- 2 Tablespoons *(6 g)* Italian seasoning
- 2 teaspoons *(6 g)* garlic powder
- 2 teaspoons *(10 g)* salt *(or to preference)*
- 1 Tablespoon *(15 ml)* avocado oil or olive oil + more *(to cook with)*

INSTRUCTIONS

1. Process the chicken breast in a food processor *(if you're not using ground chicken meat)*.

2. Mix the chicken meat with the diced apples, Italian seasoning, garlic powder, salt, and avocado oil.

3. Form 12 thin patties *(1/2-inch (1 cm) thick)* from the meat.

4. Pan fry the patties in some avocado oil *(may need to be cooked in batches)*. Place a lid over the pan to cook them faster. Check with a meat thermometer that the internal temperature of a sausage is 170 F *(77 C)*.

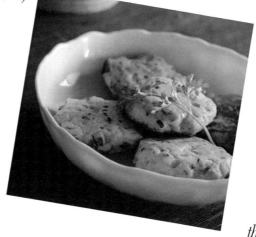

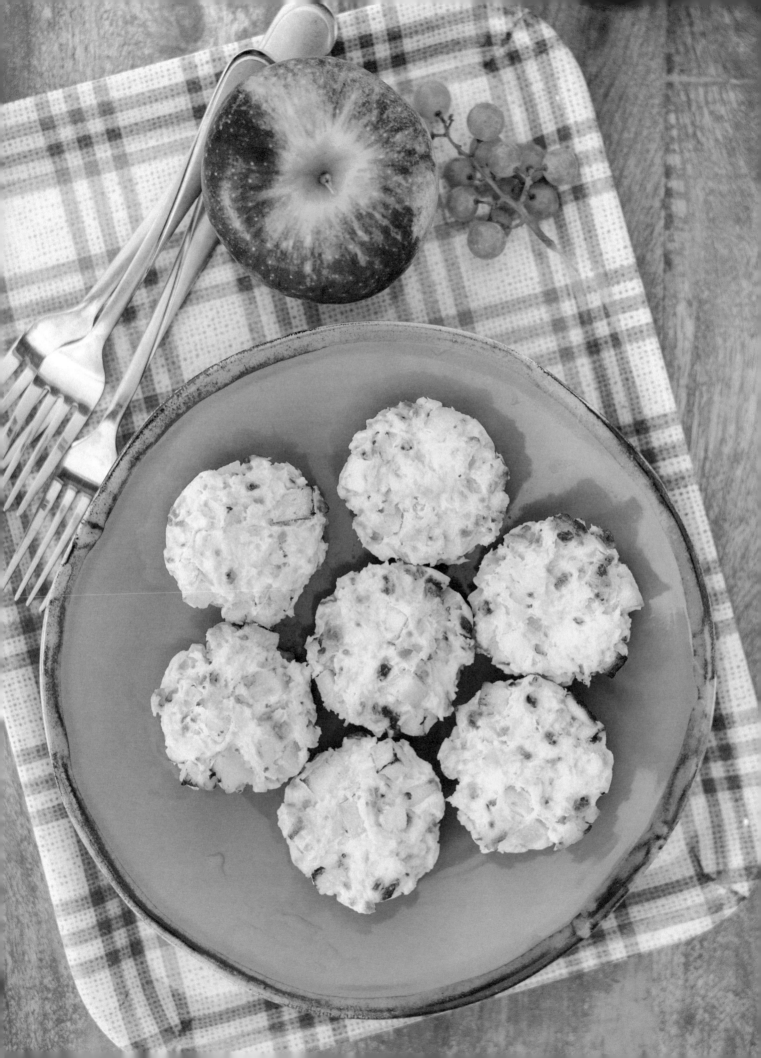

Chicken, Bacon, and Apple Mini Meatloaves

Prep Time: 15 minutes
Cook Time: 25 minutes
Total Time: 40 minutes
Yield: 4 servings
Serving Size: 3 mini meatloaves

While muffins and cupcakes don't feature much in the autoimmune protocol, muffin/cupcake pans are still useful in the kitchen! You can use them to make Easy Bacon Cups *(see Page 32 for recipe)* or to make mini meatloaves like this recipe.

Note - if you get tired of chicken meat, try switching it to beef or turkey.

INGREDIENTS

- 1 1/2 apples, diced into small cubes
- 2 chicken breasts *(approx. 1 lb or 450 g)*, minced
- 8-10 slices of bacon, cooked and crushed into bits
- 3 Tablespoons *(45 ml)* olive oil or avocado oil
- 1 teaspoon *(5 g)* salt *(more to taste)*

INSTRUCTIONS

1. Preheat oven to 400 F *(200 C)*.
2. Food process the chicken breast if it's not already minced.
3. Mix all the ingredients together in a large bowl.
4. Grease a muffin pan and form 12 mini meatloaves using the meat mixture.
5. Bake for 20-25 minutes - check with a meat thermometer that the internal temperature reaches 170 F *(77 C)*.

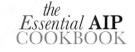

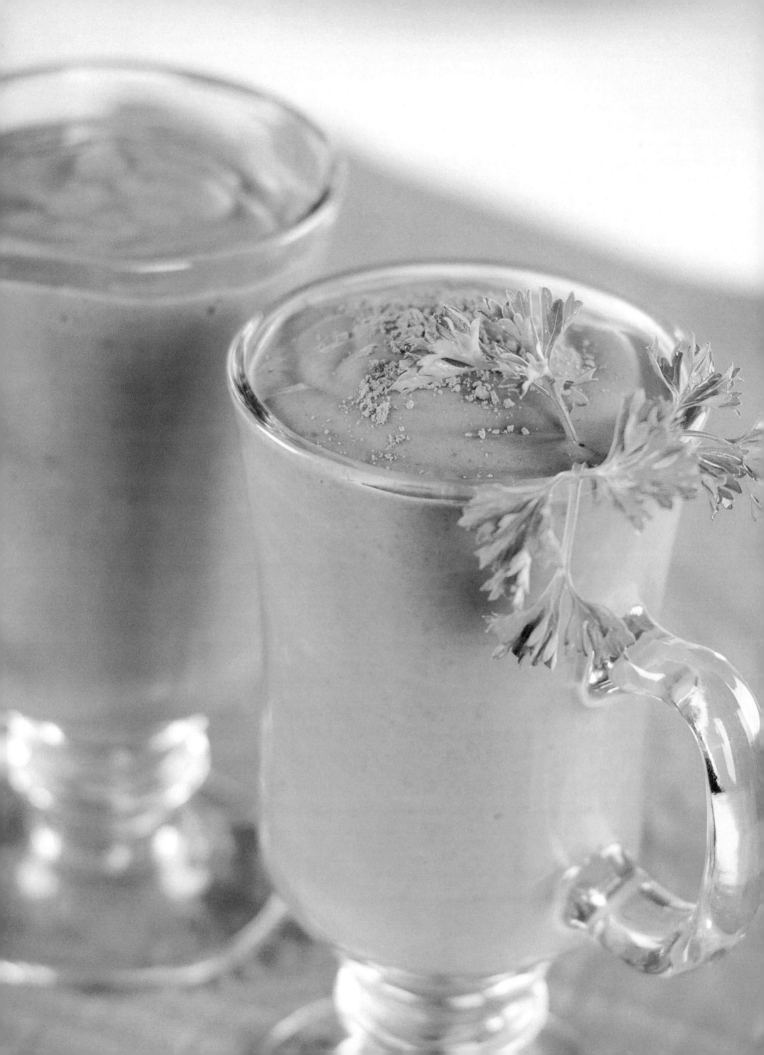

"Chocolate" Avocado Smoothie

Prep Time: 10 minutes
Cook Time: 0 minutes
Total Time: 10 minutes
Yield: 2 servings
Serving Size: 1 large glass

While chocolate and cacao powder are not considered AIP-compliant ingredients, carob powder can be a good substitute for cacao powder.

INGREDIENTS

- 1 avocado
- 2 frozen bananas
- 1/2 cup *(70 g)* frozen raspberries *(or fresh raspberries or other berries)*
- 1-2 Tablespoons *(5-10 g)* carob powder
- 2 cups *(480 ml)* coconut milk

INSTRUCTIONS

1. If you have unpeeled frozen bananas, then take the frozen bananas from the freezer and leave to thaw for 10 minutes before peeling *(or cut the skin off with a paring knife)*.

2. Place all the ingredients into a blender and blend well.

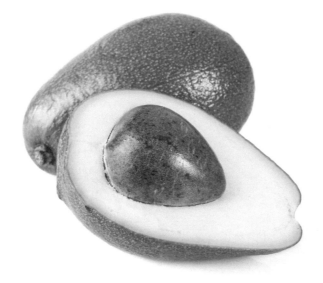

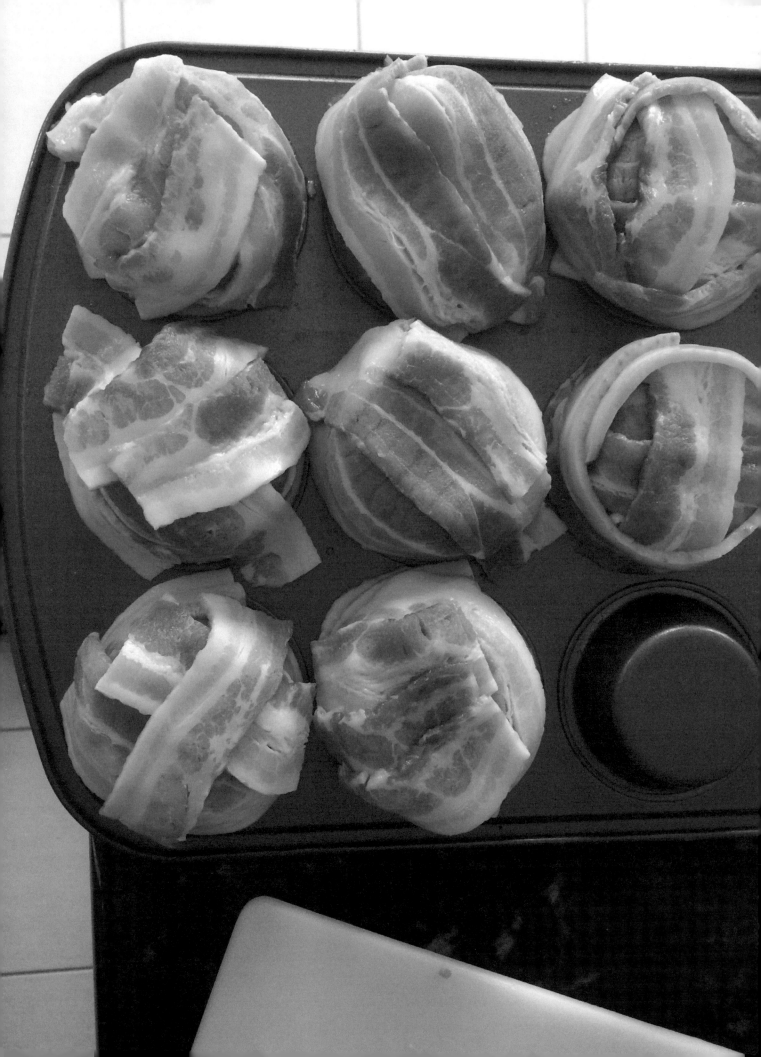

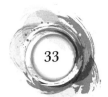

Easy Bacon Cups

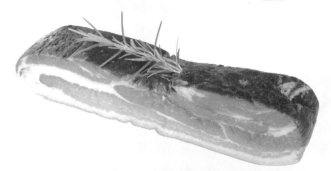

Prep Time: 15 minutes
Cook Time: 25 minutes
Total Time: 40 minutes
Yield: 3 servings
Serving Size: 2 bacon cups

While bacon is an allowed AIP ingredient, just double check the ingredients to make sure it doesn't contain any spices or artificial preservatives not permitted on AIP.

Fill these bacon cups up with some avocados, some Spinach, Mushroom, and Bacon Saute *(see Page 35 for recipe)*, or even with Chicken, Bacon, and Apple Mini Meatloaves *(see Page 28 for recipe)*.

INGREDIENTS
- 15 thin slices of bacon
- Equipment: standard nonstick metal muffin or cupcake pan

INSTRUCTIONS
1. Preheat oven to 400 F *(200 C)*.
2. Each bacon cup will require 2 and 1/2 slices of bacon, to be used as described in Step #3 below.
3. Start by turning the entire muffin/cupcake pan over, so that the side that is normally the bottom is on top. To make 1 bacon cup, place 2 half slices of bacon across the back of one of the muffin/cupcake cups, both in the same direction. Then, place another half slice across those 2, perpendicular to the direction of the first 2 half slices. Finally, wrap a whole slice of bacon tightly around the sides of the cup. The slice wrapped around the sides will help to hold the bottom pieces of bacon together.
4. Repeat Step #3 for the other 5 cups. *(You can scale this recipe to as many cups as your pan has by simply using more bacon.)*
5. Place the entire pan *(still upside-down)* into the oven and bake for 25 minutes until crispy *(place a baking tray underneath in the oven to catch any dripping bacon fat)*.
6. Cool for 5-10 minutes, and then carefully remove the bacon cups from the muffin tray.

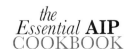

the
Essential **AIP**
COOKBOOK

Perfect Green Smoothie

Prep Time: 5 minutes
Cook Time: 0 minutes
Total Time: 5 minutes
Yield: 1 serving
Serving Size: 1 cup

INGREDIENTS

- 1 cup *(240 ml)* coconut milk
- 2 large handfuls of spinach or kale
(the amount does not need to be exact - you can also blanch them first to reduce the anti-nutrients)
- 1 Tablespoon *(15 ml)* coconut oil
- 1 ripe banana

INSTRUCTIONS

1. Place all ingredients into a blender and blend well.

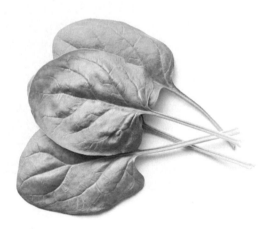

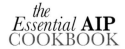

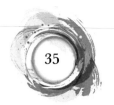

Spinach, Mushroom, Bacon Saute

Prep Time: 10 minutes
Cook Time: 0 minutes
Total Time: 10 minutes
Yield: 2 servings
Serving Size: 1 small plate

Sautes and stir-fries feature a lot in this cookbook because they're so fast and easy to make, and delicious to eat, which is important when you're focusing on healing your body. So, why not start the day with a quick saute for breakfast.

INGREDIENTS
- 4 slices of bacon, chopped
- 1/4 onion, chopped
- 3 button mushrooms, chopped
- 1 lb *(454 g)* spinach
- Salt *(to taste)*

INSTRUCTIONS
1. Add the chopped bacon into a saute pan.
2. After some of the fat has come out of the bacon, add the chopped onions into the pan and cook until the bacon is cooked and the onions are translucent.
3. Then add in the chopped mushrooms and lastly the spinach leaves.
4. Cook until spinach wilts. Add salt to taste and serve.

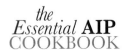

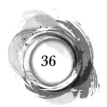

Sweet Potato Breakfast Hash

Prep Time: 10 minutes
Cook Time: 5 minutes
Total Time: 15 minutes
Yield: 2 servings
Serving Size: 1 plate

This breakfast recipe is a fantastic way to use any leftover meats from the night before. It's also a great opportunity to add in your favorite herbs.

If you don't have any leftover meats, deli meats could be used instead *(again, make sure they don't contain any spices that are non-AIP).*

INGREDIENTS
- 1 sweet potato, shredded
- 1/2 zucchini, shredded
- 1 cup leftover meat, shredded *(approx. 6 oz or 170 g)*
- 1 Tablespoon *(2 g)* fresh thyme leaves, finely chopped *(or use 1 tsp (1 g) dried thyme or use other herbs)*
- 1 Tablespoon *(15 ml)* coconut oil *(for cooking)*
- Salt *(to taste)*

INSTRUCTIONS
1. Place 1 Tablespoon of coconut oil into a frying pan on medium heat.
2. Add in the shredded sweet potato, shredded zucchini, and leftover meat. Cook until the sweet potato starts to get tender *(approx. 5 minutes).*
3. Add in the herbs and salt to taste.

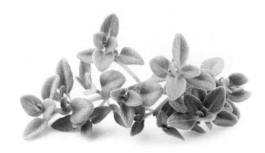

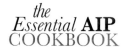

Chapter 2:
Appetizers

Autumn Butternut Squash Soup

Prep Time: 15 minutes
Cook Time: 1 hour 30 minutes
Total Time: 1 hour 45 minutes
Yield: 4 servings
Serving Size: 1 bowl

Soups are generally easy to make, and you can make them in a large batch to drink over several days. So I would encourage you to experiment with different soup recipes - I've included some basic recipes for you to start off with like this butternut squash soup.

If you don't have bone broth available as the base, you can make your own chicken stock *(just replace the bones in the bone broth recipe with a whole chicken or chicken bones)* or buy chicken stock *(again make sure they don't contain non-AIP spices)*.

INGREDIENTS
- 1 medium sized onion *(or half a large one)*, chopped
- 4 cups *(1 l)* bone broth *(see Page 183 for recipe)*
- 1 whole butternut squash
- 1 Tablespoon *(15 ml)* coconut oil
- Salt *(to taste)*
- Cinnamon *(for sprinkling)*

INSTRUCTIONS
1. Add 1 Tablespoon of coconut oil to a large pot and saute the chopped onions until they turn translucent.
2. While the onions are cooking, chop up the butternut squash *(e.g., into 1-inch or 2.5 cm thick pieces)*, remove the seeds, and then remove the skin with a sharp knife.
3. Add the chopped butternut squash and bone broth to the pot and simmer on a medium heat for 1 hour.
4. Use an immersion blender to puree the cooked veggies. *(Try to keep the end of the stick immersed in the soup to prevent too much splashing.)* If you don't have an immersion blender, then you can take the softened veggies out of the pot and place them into a blender or food processor to puree.
5. Once pureed, season the soup with salt to taste and sprinkle with cinnamon on top.

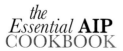

the
Essential **AIP**
COOKBOOK

Bacon Wrapped Chicken Bites

Prep Time: 10 minutes
Cook Time: 30 minutes
Total Time: 40 minutes
Yield: 4 servings
Serving Size: 6-7 pieces

While many spices have to be avoided on the autoimmune protocol, there are still some delicious flavors that can be used. In particular, garlic works well as a seasoning for many meats *(especially chicken, which can be a bit bland)*.

INGREDIENTS

- 1 large chicken breast, cut into small bites *(approx. 22-27 pieces)*
- 8-9 thin slices of bacon, cut into thirds
- 3 Tablespoons *(30 g)* garlic powder *(or 6 minced garlic cloves if preferred)*

INSTRUCTIONS

1. Preheat oven to 400 F *(200 C)* and line a baking tray with aluminum foil or parchment paper.
2. Place the garlic powder into a bowl and dip each chicken bite into the garlic powder.
3. Wrap each short bacon piece around each garlic chicken bite. Place the bacon wrapped chicken bites on the baking tray. Try to space them out so they're not touching.
4. Bake for 25-30 minutes until the bacon turns crispy. Turn the pieces after 15 minutes if you can remember.

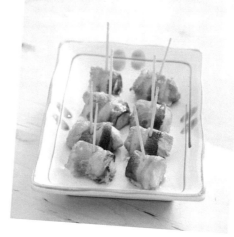

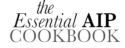

the
Essential **AIP**
COOKBOOK

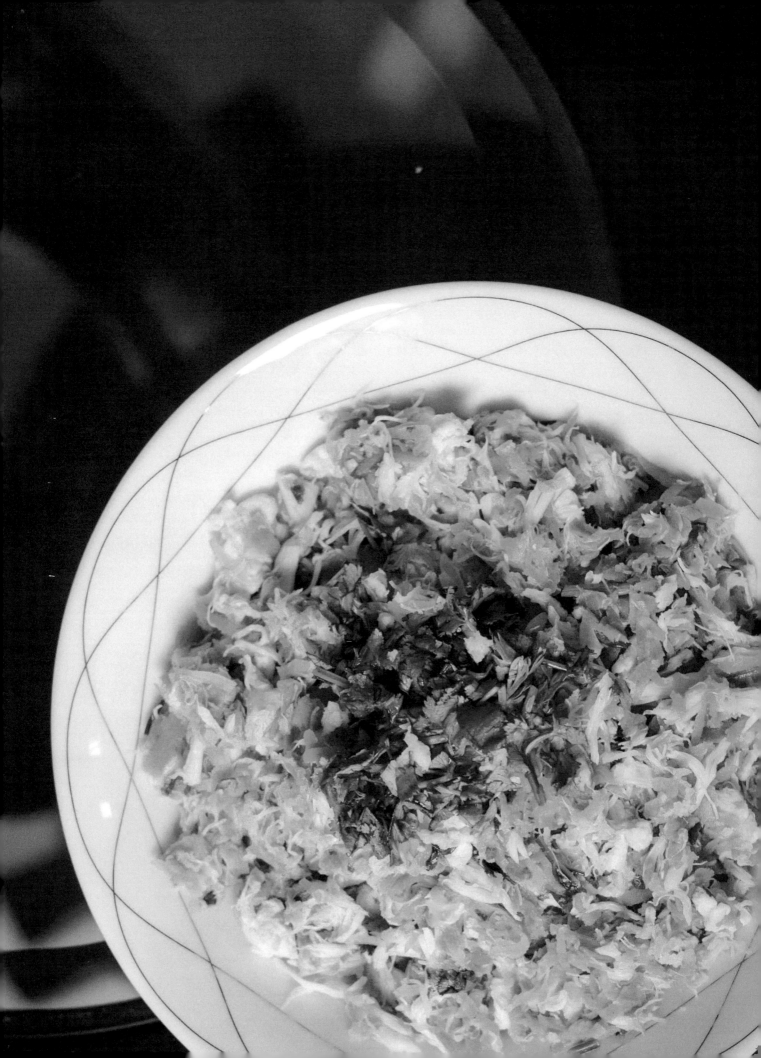

Carrot Crab Hash with Ginger and Cilantro

Prep Time: 10 minutes
Cook Time: 25 minutes
Total Time: 35 minutes
Yield: 4 servings
Serving Size: 1 small plate

This is not a "typical" recipe, but this crab hash is absolutely amazing. So, please give it a try even if you don't typically eat crab *(it's highly nutritious too)*.

INGREDIENTS

- 2 carrots, peeled and shredded
- 1 lb *(454 g)* lump crabmeat *(fresh or canned)*
- 1/4 cup *(17.5 g)* scallions *(green onions)*, chopped *(optional)*
- 1/4 cup *(15 g)* cilantro, finely chopped
- 2 cloves garlic, minced
- 2 teaspoons *(4 g)* fresh ginger, grated
- 1 Tablespoon *(15 ml)* lemon juice
- Salt *(to taste)*
- 2-4 Tablespoons *(30-60 ml)* coconut oil

INSTRUCTIONS

1. Place 2-4 Tablespoons of coconut oil into a frying pan *(or a saucepan)* and saute the carrots on medium-high heat until they start to soften *(add more coconut oil as the carrots soak it up)*. This takes approx. 15 minutes.
2. Add in the crabmeat and scallions and saute for 5-10 minutes more.
3. Lastly, add the cilantro, garlic, ginger, lemon juice, and salt to taste. Saute for a few minutes more to combine the flavors.
4. Serve immediately.

SUBSTITUTIONS

- Chicken breast *(finely diced)* can be used instead of crabmeat, but you should cook it separately before adding to the carrots.
- Apple cider vinegar can be used instead of lemon juice.

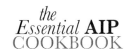

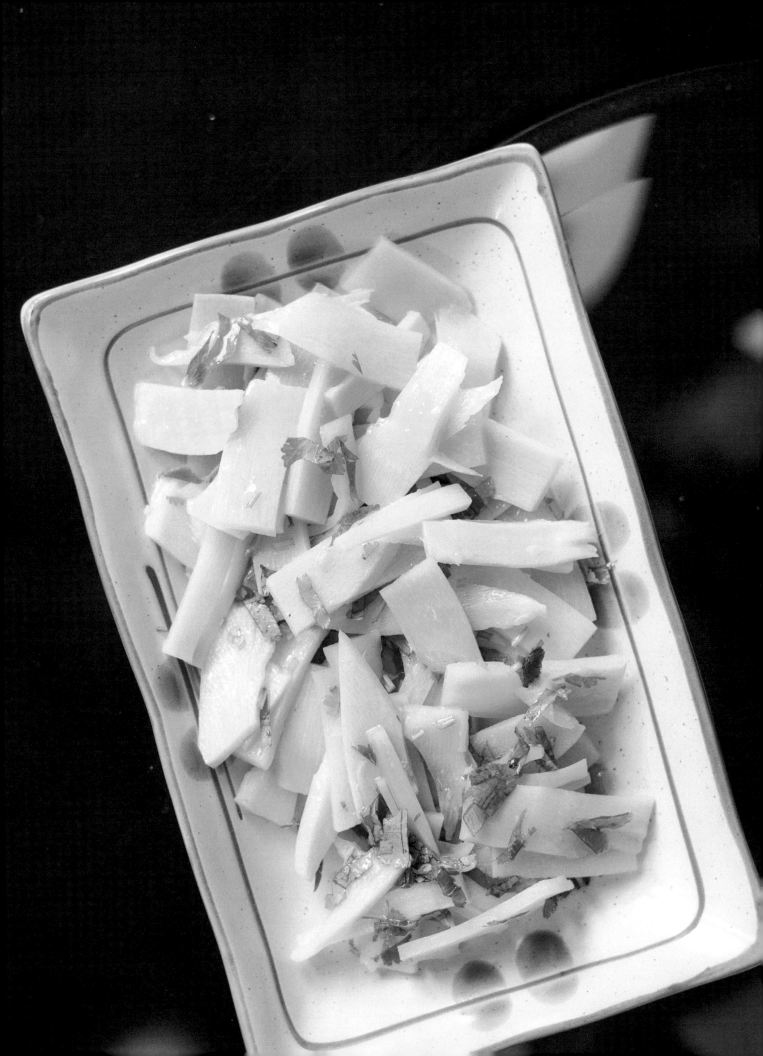

Chinese Bamboo Salad

Prep Time: 5 minutes
Cook Time: 0 minutes
Total Time: 5 minutes
Yield: 2 servings
Serving Size: 1/2 cup

This is a really easy Chinese dish to recreate at home. You can usually find canned bamboo shoots in Asian supermarkets as well as some larger regular supermarkets. And if bamboo shoots are too difficult to find, then use lightly boiled/steamed asparagus instead.

INGREDIENTS
- 1 8-ounce *(227 g)* can sliced bamboo shoots
- 2 Tablespoons *(4 g)* cilantro, finely chopped
- 1 Tablespoon *(15 ml)* olive oil
- Salt *(to taste)*

INSTRUCTIONS
1. Drain the bamboo shoots and toss with the cilantro, olive oil, and salt.

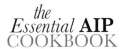

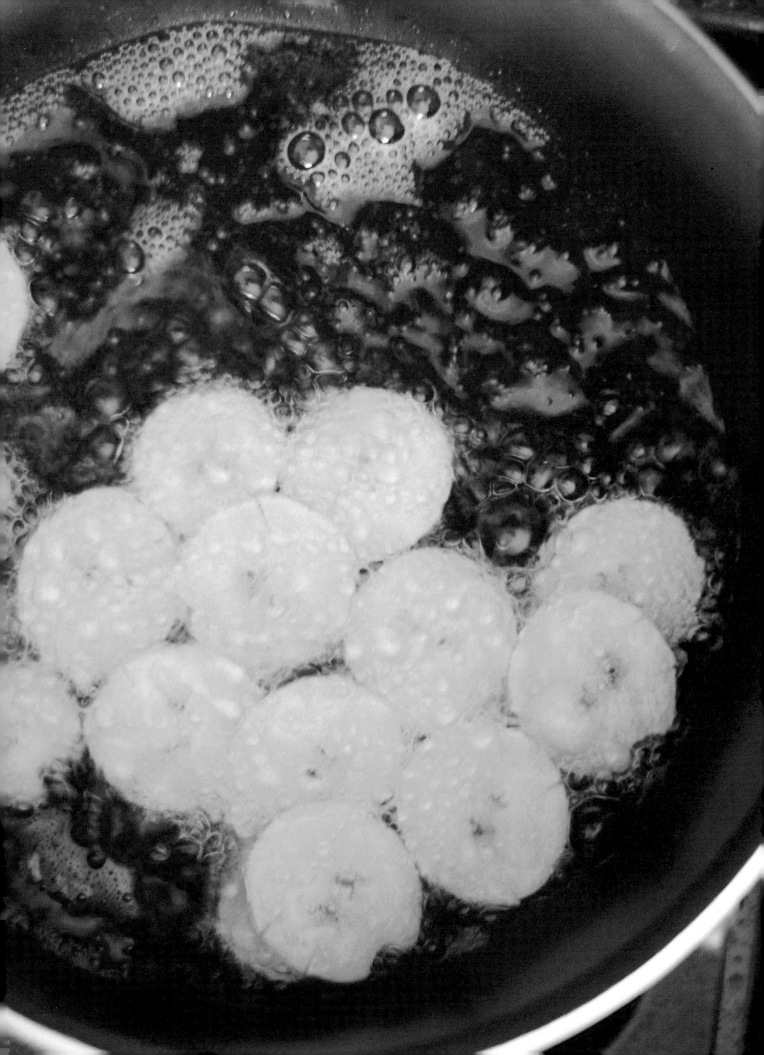

Coconut Plantain Chips

Prep Time: 15 minutes
Cook Time: 30 minutes
Total Time: 45 minutes
Yield: 2 servings
Serving Size: 1 small bowl

These plantain chips are a little addictive and take a bit of effort to make, but if you want a good snack, this is where to start. They're also a great way to start a meal.

INGREDIENTS

- 2 plantains *(green or ripe)*, peeled and sliced as thin as possible
- Approx. 1/2 cup *(120 ml)* coconut oil *(depends how big the saucepan is)*
- Salt *(to taste)*

INSTRUCTIONS

1. Place the coconut oil into a saucepan so that it's approx. 1/4-inch deep *(or use a deep fat fryer)*.
2. Heat up the oil for 3-4 minutes on a medium heat.
3. Drop in each thin slice of plantain one by one into the oil so they're not overlapping.
4. Use a perforated spoon to get the slices out as soon as they turn golden.
5. Repeat until all the slices are fried.
6. Dust with salt to taste and mix well without breaking any of the chips!

SUBSTITUTIONS:

- Use sweet potatoes instead of plantains to make sweet potato chips.
- Bananas can be used instead of plantains.

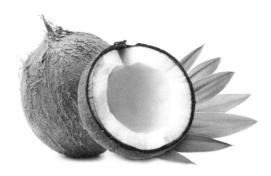

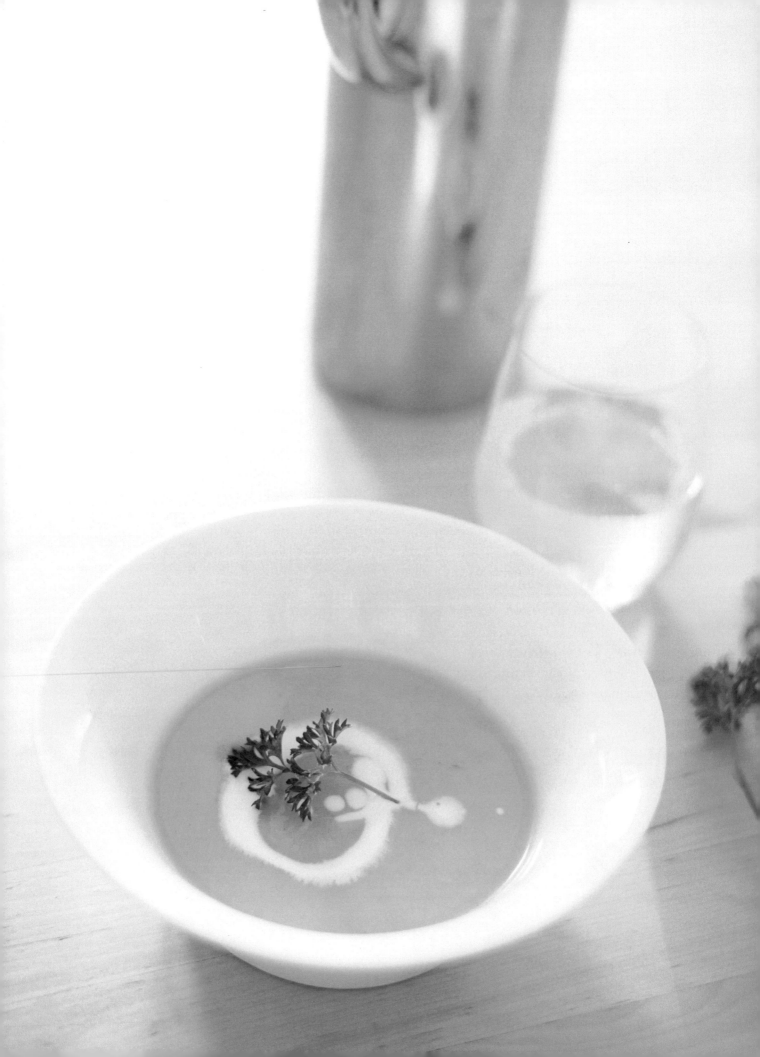

Creamy Leek and Cauliflower Soup

Prep Time: 10 minutes
Cook Time: 1 hour
Total Time: 1 hour 10 minutes
Yield: 4 servings
Serving Size: 1 cup

Cauliflower is really cool. You can use it to make "rice" dishes *(there are a couple recipes in this cookbook)*, to make porridge, or you can use it to replicate potatoes. In soups, this comes in very handy. This soup is a great Fall/Winter soup. The leek adds a lot of flavor, and the cauliflower provides the thick texture.

INGREDIENTS

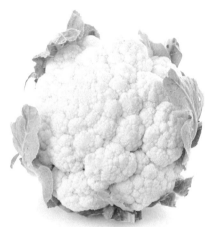

- 1 large leek *(approx. 225 g)*
- 1/2 cauliflower *(approx. 280 g)*
- 1/2 cup *(120 ml)* coconut cream, warmed
- 3 cups *(720 ml)* chicken or bone broth *(see Page 183 for recipe)*
- Salt *(to taste)*
- Bacon bits *(optional)*
- 2 Tablespoons *(30 ml)* coconut cream *(for drizzling)*

INSTRUCTIONS

1. Cut the cauliflower and leek into small pieces.
2. Place the cauliflower and leek into a large pot with the chicken or bone broth *(or use a pressure cooker)*.
3. Cover the pot and simmer for 1 hour or until tender.
4. Use an immersion blender to puree the vegetables to create a smooth soup. *(If you don't have an immersion blender, you can take the vegetables out, let cool briefly, puree in a normal blender, and then put back into the pot.)*
5. Add in the coconut cream and salt to taste and mix well.
6. Drizzle with some coconut cream and top with bacon bits for garnish.

SUBSTITUTIONS

- Onion can be used instead of leek *(use 1 small white or yellow onion)*.
- Coconut cream can be omitted.

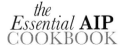

the
Essential **AIP**
COOKBOOK

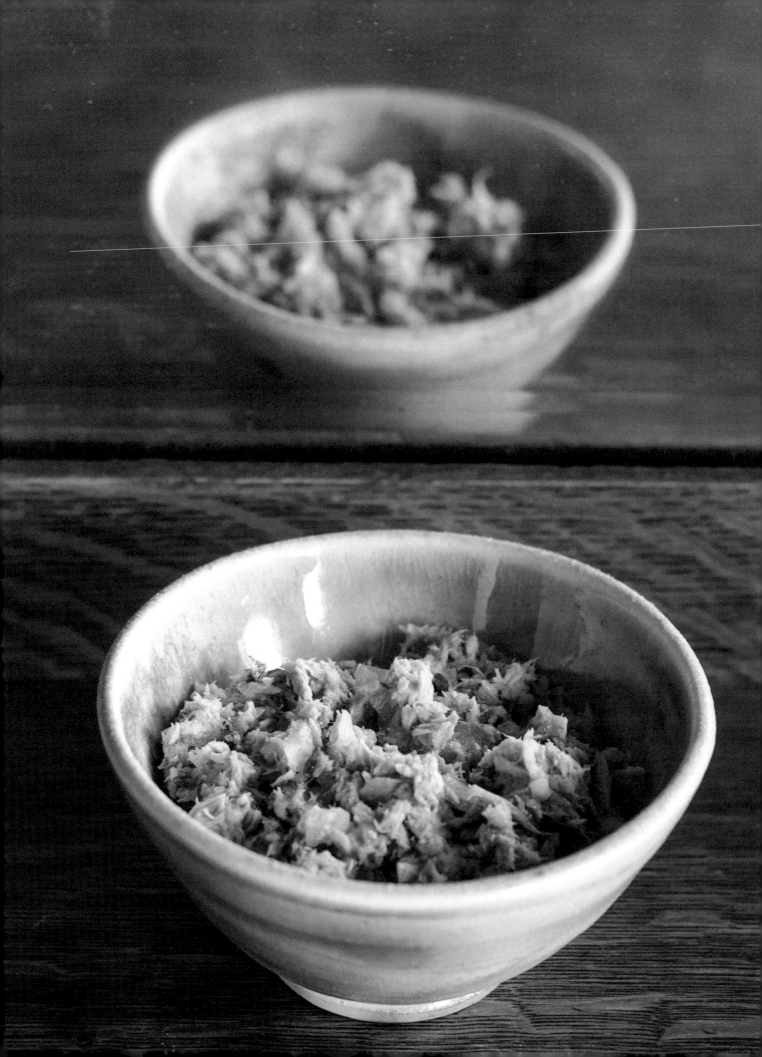

Easy Tuna Salad

Prep Time: 15 minutes
Cook Time: 0 minutes
Total Time: 15 minutes
Yield: 2 servings
Serving Size: 1 small plate

Getting more seafood into your diet is always a good idea as it's highly nutritious, and eating more tuna is one of the easiest ways as you can generally find canned tuna even in areas far from the sea.

INGREDIENTS

- 1/4 cucumber, peeled and diced finely
- 2 5-oz *(284 g)* cans of tuna
- 1-2 stalks of celery, diced finely
- 2 Tablespoons *(30 ml)* olive oil
- 1 clove garlic, minced
- 3 Tablespoons *(45 g)* finely chopped parsley
- 1/2 Tablespoon *(7 ml)* lemon juice
- Salt *(to taste)*

INSTRUCTIONS

1. Flake the tuna and chop the cucumber into small pieces.
2. Mix the tuna together with the chopped cucumber, celery, olive oil, garlic, parsley, and lemon juice. Add salt to taste and combine well.

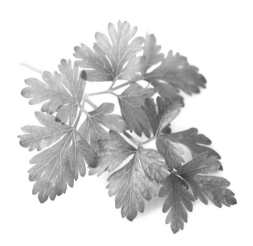

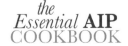
the Essential **AIP**
COOKBOOK

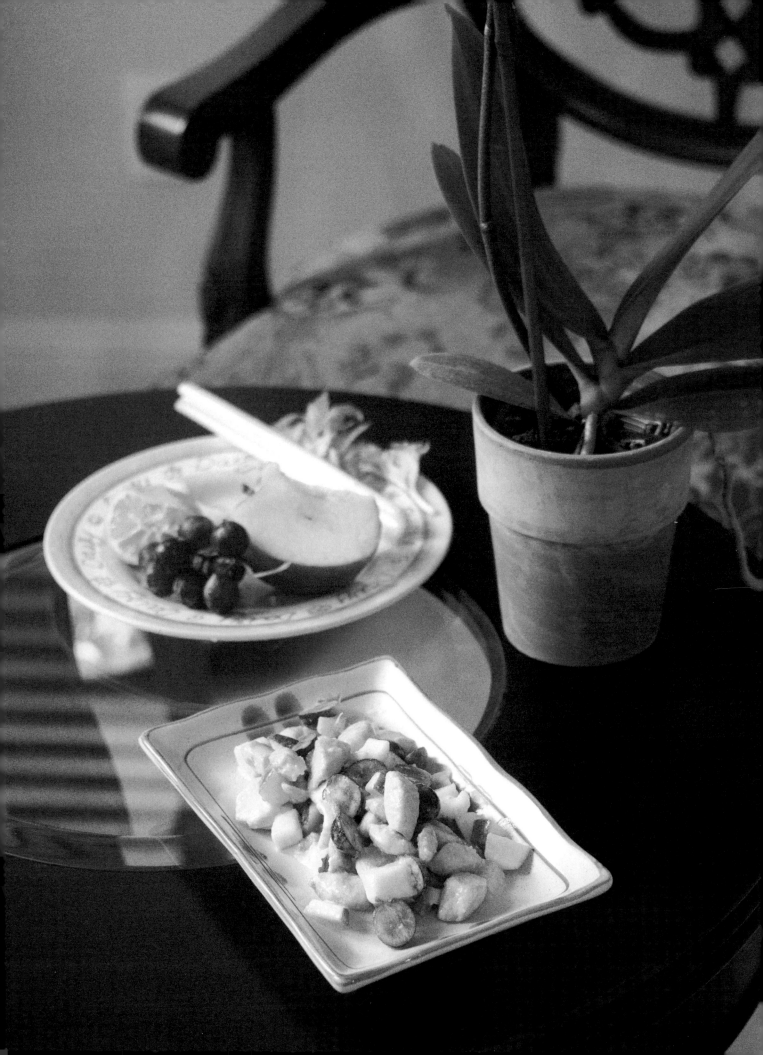

Grape and Apple Chicken Salad

Prep Time: 10 minutes
Cook Time: 10 minutes
Total Time: 20 minutes
Yield: 2 servings
Serving Size: 1 small plate

Salads are so easy to make and so refreshing to enjoy - this one is no different! The apples and grapes add the sweetness and the crunch in this simple salad.

INGREDIENTS

- 1 chicken breast, diced
- Coconut oil *(to cook chicken in)*
- 25 grapes, halved
- 1/2 gala apple, diced
- 1 stalk of celery, diced
- 1/4 cup *(60 ml)* coconut milk *(from a can shaken and at room temperature)*
- Salt *(to taste)*

INSTRUCTIONS

1. Saute the diced chicken breast in coconut oil until cooked.
2. Wait for the chicken to cool then add it to the halved grapes, diced apple, and diced celery in a large bowl. Add in the coconut milk and salt to taste.
3. Toss well.

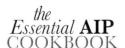

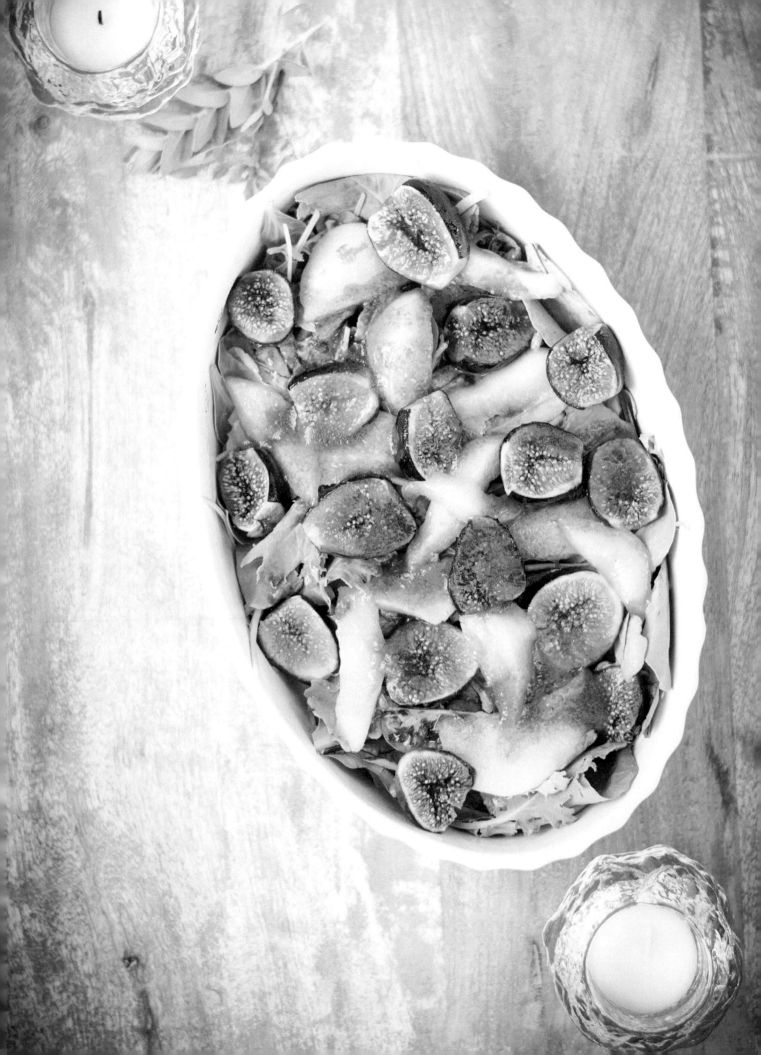

Honey Roasted Pear and Fig Salad With Ginger Balsamic Vinaigrette

Prep Time: 10 minutes
Cook Time: 15 minutes
Total Time: 25 minutes
Yield: 4 servings
Serving Size: 1 plate

INGREDIENTS

- 8 figs, cut off stem from each side and halved
- 1 pear, peeled and sliced
- 1 Tablespoon *(15 ml)* coconut oil
- 1/2 Tablespoon *(10.5 g)* honey
- Salad greens

For the Vinaigrette:

- 1 Tablespoon *(21 g)* honey
- 3 Tablespoons *(45 ml)* balsamic vinegar
- 1 Tablespoon *(5 g)* ginger
- 1/2 cup *(120 ml)* olive oil *(or avocado oil)*

INSTRUCTIONS

1. Preheat oven to 400 F *(200 C)*.
2. Melt the coconut oil and honey slightly and coat the pear slices and fig halves with the mixture. Place onto a baking tray and bake for 15 minutes.
3. Place all the vinaigrette ingredients into a blender and blend well.
4. To serve, place the baked figs and pear slices on top of the salad greens. Drizzle the vinaigrette over the top.

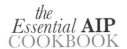

Pan-Fried Apricot Tuna Salad Bites

Prep Time: 15 minutes
Cook Time: 5 minutes
Total Time: 20 minutes
Yield: 5 servings
Serving Size: 2 halves

These are perfect for parties or when you have guests come over.

INGREDIENTS

- 5 apricots, sliced in half and stones removed
- 2 5-oz *(284 g)* cans of tuna, flaked
- 2 Tablespoons *(4 g)* thyme leaves, diced
- 2 Tablespoons *(30 ml)* olive oil *(or mayo)*
- Sea salt *(to taste)*
- Coconut oil *(to pan-fry the apricot halves in)*
- 5 blueberries, sliced in half

INSTRUCTIONS

1. Place coconut oil into a frying pan and pan-fry the apricot halves cut-face down so they're slightly browned. Alternatively, you can grill the apricot halves instead.
2. In a bowl, mix together the tuna, thyme leaves, olive oil, and sea salt to taste.
3. Use a spoon to pile mounds of the tuna mixture on top of the apricot halves.
4. Top each tuna apricot bite with half a blueberry.

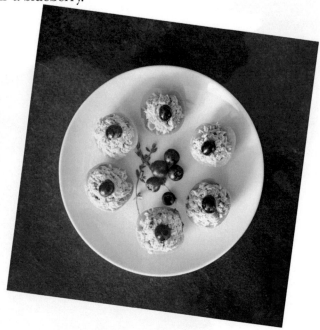

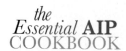

Lemon Fried Avocado Slices

Prep Time: 5 minutes
Cook Time: 5 minutes
Total Time: 10 minutes
Yield: 2 servings
Serving Size: 6 slices

These are so easy and delicious to make - just be careful not to burn them as they brown quickly. This recipe is especially good for avocados you've bought that aren't quite ripe yet - this will softened them up and make them more tasty.

INGREDIENTS

- 1 ripe avocado *(not too soft)*, cut into slices
- 1 Tablespoon *(15 ml)* coconut oil
- 1 Tablespoon *(15 ml)* lemon juice
- Salt *(to taste) (or lemon salt)*

INSTRUCTIONS

1. Pour the lemon juice over the avocado slices.
2. Add the coconut oil to a frying pan. Place the avocado slices into the oil gently.
3. Fry the avocado slices *(turning gently)* so that all sides are slightly browned.
4. Add salt to taste and serve warm.

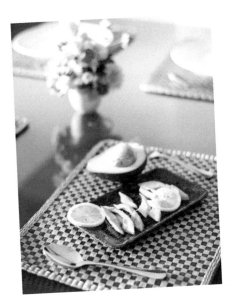

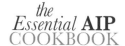

Refreshing Mint Cucumber Melon Soup

Prep Time: 15 minutes
Cook Time: 0 minutes
Total Time: 15 minutes
Yield: 4 servings
Serving Size: 1 bowl

This soup is raw and best served chilled.

INGREDIENTS
- 1 long cucumber, chilled, peeled, and chopped into chunks
- 1/4 -1/2 honeydew melon *(depending on sweetness)*, chilled, and chopped into chunks
- Approx. 10 mint leaves

INSTRUCTIONS
1. Blend everything together really well.
2. Garnish with a mint leaf.

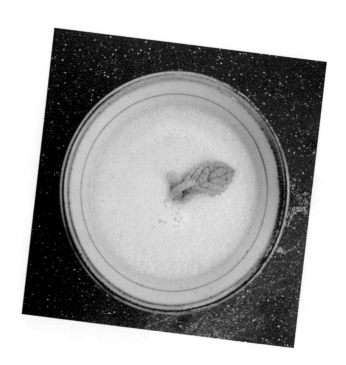

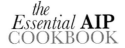

Simple Coleslaw Salad

Prep Time: 15 minutes
Cook Time: 0 minutes
Total Time: 15 minutes
Yield: 2 servings
Serving Size: 1 cup

Most coleslaw recipes use mayo, which contains eggs, but this recipe uses an olive oil-based mixture instead.

INGREDIENTS

- 1 head of cabbage *(green or purple)*, thinly shredded *(use food processor shredding attachment)*
- 2 carrots, peeled and thinly shredded
- 1/4 onion, peeled and thinly shredded
- 1 cup *(240 ml)* olive oil
- 1 Tablespoon *(21 g)* raw honey
- 1/4 cup *(60 ml)* apple cider vinegar
- 1 teaspoon *(3 g)* garlic powder
- Salt *(to taste)*

INSTRUCTIONS

1. Squeeze out excess water from the shredded vegetables and add them to a large bowl.

2. In a separate bowl, mix together the olive oil, honey, vinegar, garlic powder, and salt.

3. Add the dressing to the vegetables and mix well.

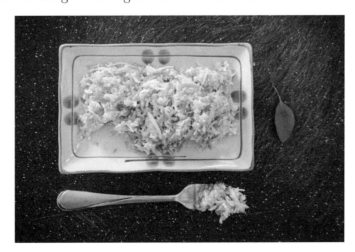

Splendid Strawberry Spinach Salad

Prep Time: 10 minutes
Cook Time: 0 minutes
Total Time: 10 minutes
Yield: 4 servings
Serving Size: 1 small bowl

INGREDIENTS

- 2 ounces *(57 g or approx. 4-6 handfuls)* baby spinach leaves, washed
- 10 medium-sized strawberries

For the Dressing:

- 3 strawberries
- 1 teaspoon *(5 ml)* raw honey
- 1/3 cup *(80 ml)* olive oil
- 1 Tablespoon *(15 ml)* apple cider vinegar

INSTRUCTIONS

1. Slice up the 10 strawberries and add to a large bowl with the spinach.
2. Place all the dressing ingredients into a blender and blend well. Toss the dressing with the salad.

SUBSTITUTIONS

- Other berries can be used instead of strawberries
- Other sugars can be used instead of raw honey.
- Balsamic vinegar can be used instead of apple cider vinegar.

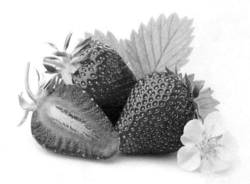

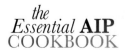

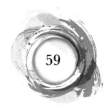

Thai Lemongrass Shrimp Soup

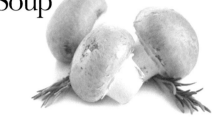

Prep Time: 10 minutes
Cook Time: 30 minutes
Total Time: 40 minutes
Yield: 4 servings
Serving Size: 1 bowl

This soup is another great way to get more seafood into your diet. Plus, it's delicious with the lemongrass, ginger, fish sauce, lime juice, and cilantro all adding to the flavor.

INGREDIENTS

- 16 large shrimp *(approx. 1 lb (454 g))*
- 2-3 cups *(480-720 ml)* coconut cream *(or alternatively use the top layer of cream from a refrigerated can of coconut milk)*
- 4 cups *(1 l)* chicken broth or bone broth *(see Page 183 for recipe)*
- 3 large button mushrooms, sliced
- 1 lemongrass stalk, split down the center and then chopped into 2-inch long chunks
- 1 teaspoon *(2 g)* ginger, freshly grated *(traditional recipe uses thin slices of galangal)*
- 3 Tablespoons *(45 ml)* fish sauce
- Juice from 1/2 a lime
- Salt *(to taste)*
- 2 Tablespoons *(4 g)* cilantro, finely chopped *(for garnish)*

INSTRUCTIONS

1. Heat the broth in a medium-sized pot and add in the mushrooms, lemongrass, ginger, fish sauce, and lime juice.
2. Simmer for 10 minutes.
3. Add in the coconut cream and simmer for another 10 minutes until the coconut cream mixes in well.
4. Taste the broth and add in salt to taste. Add in more fish sauce, lime juice, or coconut cream depending on how you like the soup.
5. Add in the shrimp and simmer until the shrimp is cooked.
6. Serve immediately with the cilantro as garnish.

SUBSTITUTIONS

- Chicken breast cut into small chunks can be used instead of shrimp.
- Instead of button mushrooms, you can use straw or shiitake mushrooms.

the
Essential **AIP**
COOKBOOK

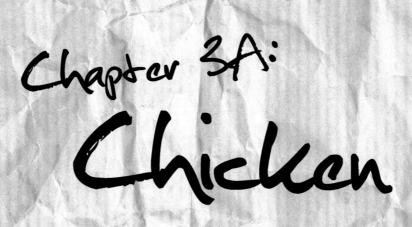

Chapter 3A:
Chicken

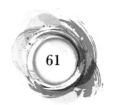

Grilled Chicken Drumsticks with Garlic Marinade

Prep Time: 10 minutes
Cook Time: 20 minutes
Total Time: 30 minutes
Yield: 2 servings
Serving Size: 3 drumsticks

Enjoy with a side of Creamy Mashed Sweet Potatoes *(see Page 136 for recipe)*.

INGREDIENTS

- 6 chicken drumsticks
- 1 cup *(240 ml)* olive oil
- 7 cloves garlic
- 1 Tablespoon *(10 g)* garlic powder
- Juice from 1/2 lemon
- 1/2 Tablespoon *(7.5 g)* salt

INSTRUCTIONS

1. To make the marinade for the chicken, place the olive oil, garlic, garlic powder, lemon juice, and salt into a blender or food processor and puree.

2. Rub the chicken drumsticks in the marinade.

3. Grill the chicken drumsticks *(use a low heat)*. Pour any leftover marinade over the chicken as it's grilling.

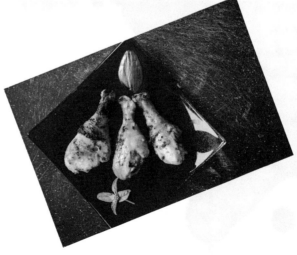

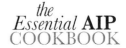

the *Essential* **AIP** COOKBOOK

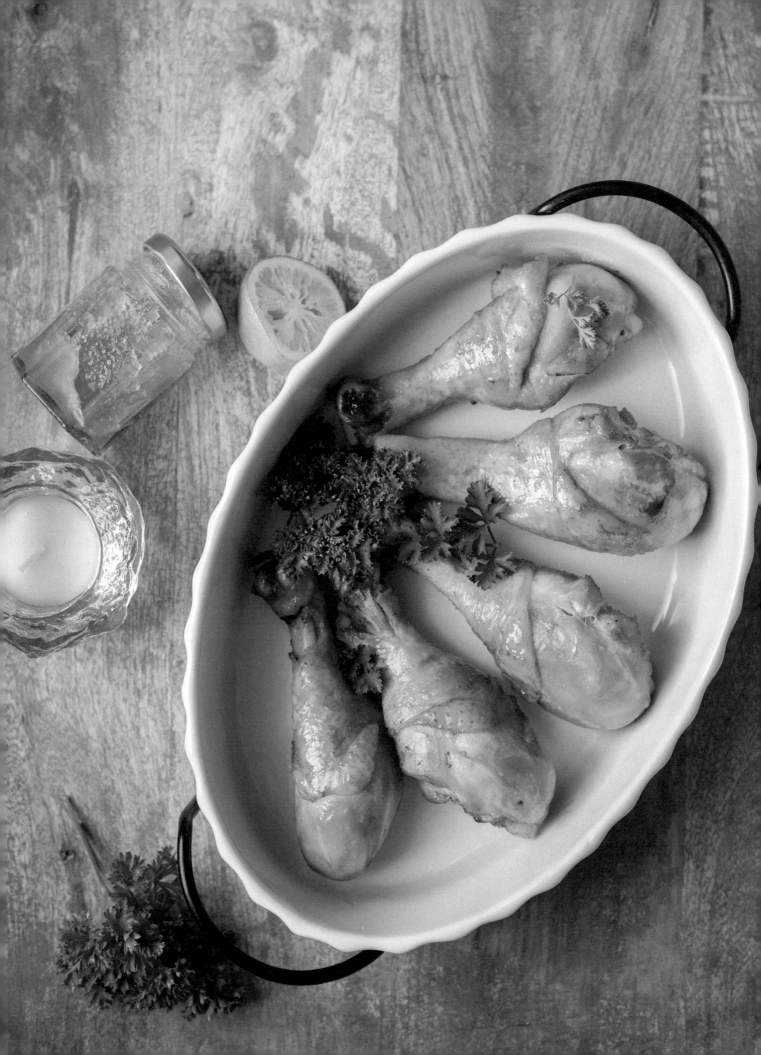

Honey Glazed Chicken Drumsticks

Prep Time: 10 minutes
Cook Time: 30 minutes
Total Time: 40 minutes
Yield: 2 servings
Serving Size: 4 drumsticks

This dish combines a lot of flavors - salty with sweet with sour - which makes it very tasty. Plus of course, it's really easy to make!

INGREDIENTS

- 8 chicken drumsticks
- 3 Tablespoons *(45 g)* salt
- 1 1/2 Tablespoons *(31.5 g)* raw honey
- 1/2 cup *(120 ml)* coconut aminos
- Juice from 1 lime

INSTRUCTIONS

1. Preheat oven to 400 F *(200 C)*.
2. Dissolve the salt into a pot of cold water. Place the chicken drumsticks in the salted water and bring to the boil - then boil for 5 minutes.
3. Make the honey sauce by mixing together the honey, coconut aminos, and lime juice. Save 1/4 of the sauce for serving.
4. Coat the boiled chicken drumsticks in the honey sauce and place on a baking tray.
5. Bake for 10 minutes and turn them.
6. Bake for 10-20 more minutes until skin becomes crispier.
7. Drizzle the sauce you saved onto the drumsticks and serve.

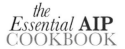

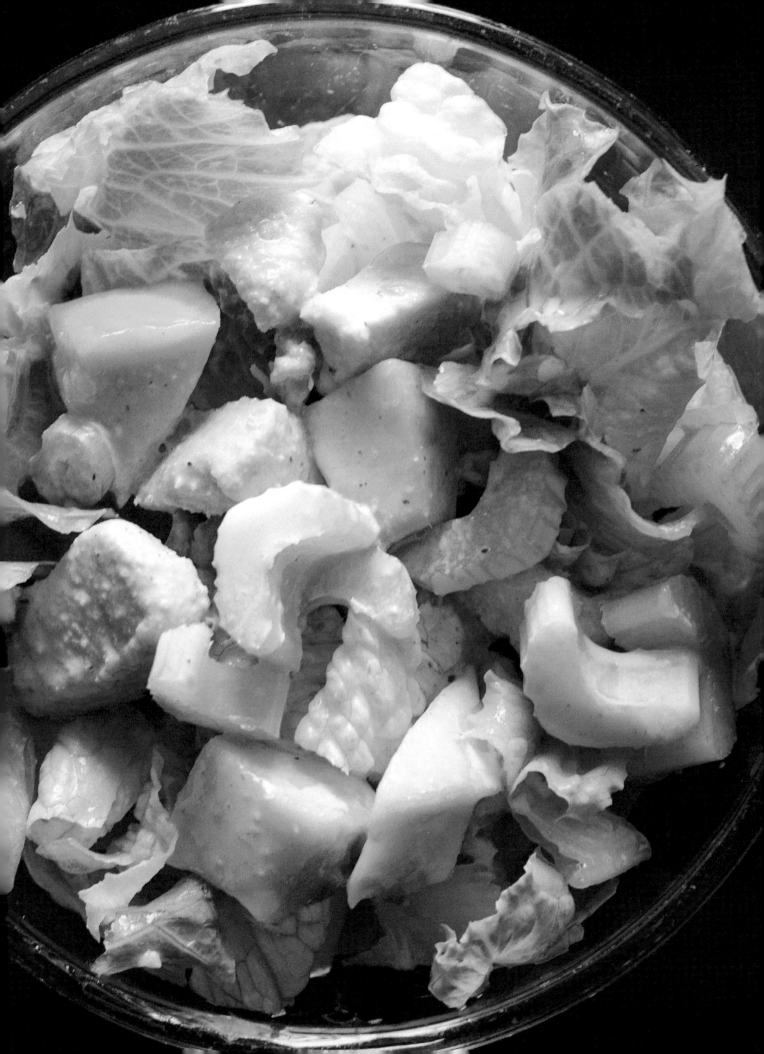

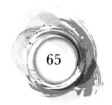

Mango and Chicken Salad with Coconut Caesar Dressing

Prep Time: 10 minutes
Cook Time: 10 minutes
Total Time: 20 minutes
Yield: 2 servings
Serving Size: 1 bowl

INGREDIENTS

- 2 chicken breasts, diced
- Coconut oil *(to cook with)*
- 1 head of romaine lettuce, washed and chopped
- 1 mango, peeled and diced

For the Salad Dressing:

- 1/2 cup *(120 ml)* coconut cream *(cream from the top of a refrigerated can of coconut milk)*
- 2 Tablespoons *(30 ml)* coconut oil
- 2 cloves garlic *(or 1/4 teaspoon (0.8 g) garlic powder)*
- Salt *(to taste)*

INSTRUCTIONS

1. Add 2 Tablespoons of coconut oil into a frying pan or skillet. Cook the diced chicken in the frying pan. Season with salt to taste.
2. Blend the coconut cream, coconut oil, garlic, and salt to make the salad dressing.
3. Toss the romaine lettuce, cooked diced chicken, and diced mango with the salad dressing.

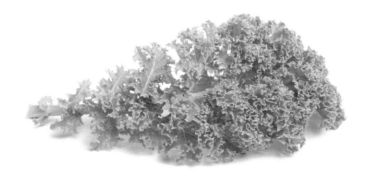

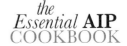

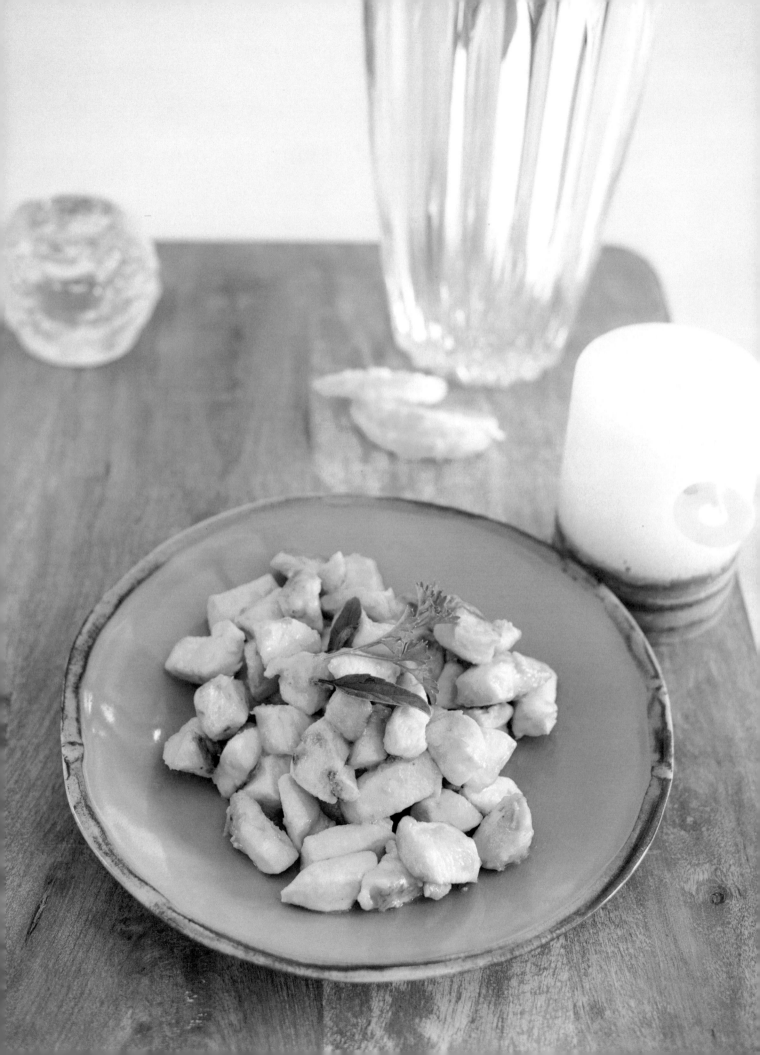

Orange Chicken Stir-Fry

Prep Time: 5 minutes
Cook Time: 10 minutes
Total Time: 15 minutes
Yield: 2 servings
Serving Size: 1 plate

Enjoy with some Ginger and Garlic Bok Choy Stir-Fry *(see Page 141 for recipe)*.

INGREDIENTS

- 2 Tablespoons *(30 ml)* avocado oil or coconut oil
- 2 chicken breasts, diced
- 1/2 teaspoon *(2.5 g)* salt
- 1 navel orange, peeled
- 1 Tablespoon *(15 ml)* coconut aminos
- 1 teaspoon *(1.7 g)* fresh ginger
- 4 cloves garlic, peeled

INSTRUCTIONS

1. Stir-fry the diced chicken breast in the avocado oil – sprinkle the salt on it.

2. Make the orange sauce by blending the navel orange with the coconut aminos, ginger, and garlic.

3. Once the chicken starts to brown, add in half the sauce.

4. Stir-fry on high heat until the liquid disappears.

5. Serve with the rest of the sauce.

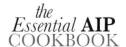

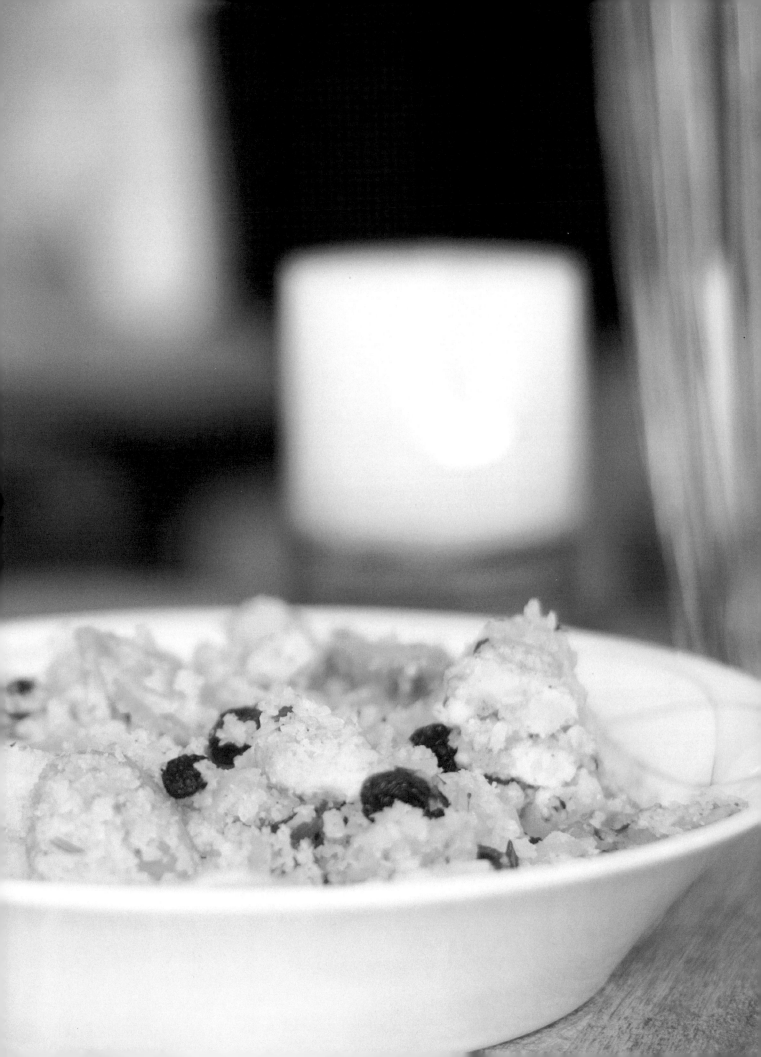

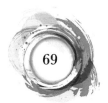

Pineapple Fried "Rice"

Prep Time: 15 minutes
Cook Time: 25 minutes
Total Time: 40 minutes
Servings: 2 servings
Yield: 1 large bowl

INGREDIENTS

- 1 head of cauliflower, broken into florets
- 1 large chicken breast, sliced thin
- 1/4 cup *(28.75 g)* raisins
- 1 cup *(165 g)* of pineapple chunks *(can be frozen)*
- 1/2 small carrot *(25 g)*, sliced
- 1/2 onion *(55 g)*, diced
- 1/4 cup *(15 g)* cilantro, finely chopped
- 1 green onion *(15 g)*, finely chopped
- Coconut oil *(to cook with)*
- Salt *(to taste)*

INSTRUCTIONS

1. Dry the cauliflower florets and food process the cauliflower into a rice-like texture. Squeeze out excess water.
2. Add 2 Tablespoons of coconut oil to a large pan on medium heat, add the chopped onions to the pan and saute them until they turn translucent.
3. Add 2 Tablespoons of coconut oil to another pan and saute the chicken breasts.
4. Add in the cauliflower "rice" to the pan with the onions.
5. Once the chicken is pretty much cooked, add the pineapples and carrots to the chicken. When the carrots have softened, add the chicken, carrots, and pineapples to the cauliflower pot.
6. Add salt to taste and keep cooking until the cauliflower is soft and the pineapples are juicy *(approx. 5-10 minutes)*. Stir frequently to prevent anything sticking to the bottom of the pan.
7. Add in the cilantro and green onions and serve.

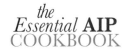

Pressure Cooker Chicken Stew

Prep Time: 15 minutes
Cook Time: 35 minutes
Total Time: 50 minutes
Yield: 2 servings
Serving Size: 1 bowl

Sometimes it can be really comforting to have a bowl of chicken stew. This is especially true during the winter months. If you don't have a pressure cooker, don't worry, you can use a slow cooker or a regular pot on the stove for this recipe.

And if you have time, also make a large batch of Rosemary Roasted Vegetables *(see Page 147 for recipe)* to enjoy this stew with.

INGREDIENTS

- 2 chicken breasts *(approx. 1 lb or 454 g)*, diced
- 4 cups *(1 l)* chicken broth or water or bone broth *(see Page 183 for recipe)*
- 2 small carrots, chopped
- 3 stalks of celery, chopped
- 1 teaspoon *(5 ml)* coconut aminos
- 1/2 Tablespoon *(1 g)* fresh thyme leaves *(or use 1/2 tsp (0.5 g) dried thyme)*
- 1/2 cup *(16 g)* parsley, chopped and divided *(save half for when you're serving)*
- 1 Tablespoon *(7 g)* unflavored gelatin powder *(optional)*
- Salt *(to taste)*
- Arrowroot flour/powder *(for thickening)*

INSTRUCTIONS

1. Place the diced chicken breasts, chicken broth, chopped carrots, chopped celery, coconut aminos, thyme, and half the parsley into the pressure cooker pot.
2. If you're adding in gelatin, then stir it in until it dissolves.
3. Set the pressure cooker on high pressure for 35 minutes. When ready, follow your pressure cooker's instructions for releasing the pressure safely.
4. Add salt to taste and sprinkle in the rest of the chopped parsley.
5. If you want to thicken the stew, then mix 2 Tablespoons *(16 g)* of arrowroot flour in 1/4 cup *(60 ml)* of cold water and pour the mixture into the hot stew. Stir and serve immediately.

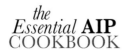

Slow Cooker Apple Honey Chicken Drumsticks

Prep Time: 5 minutes
Cook Time: 6 hours
Total Time: 6 hours 5 minutes
Yield: 2 servings
Serving Size: 4 drumsticks

Serve with a large plate of Easy Bacon Brussels Sprouts *(see Page 137 for recipe)* for a delicious dinner.

INGREDIENTS

- 3 apples, peeled and diced
- 1 Tablespoon *(21 g)* honey
- 8 chicken drumsticks
- 1 teaspoon *(5 g)* salt
- 1/2 teaspoon *(1 g)* cinnamon *(optional)*

INSTRUCTIONS

1. Place everything into a slow cooker and mix well so that the honey and salt coat the chicken drumsticks.
2. Cook on low for 5-6 hours until chicken is tender.
3. Serve the chicken drumsticks with the now mushy apple sauce.

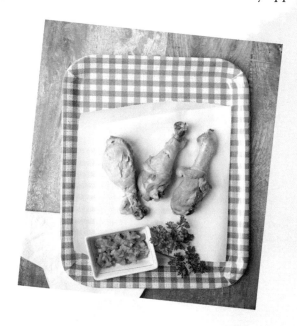

Slow Cooker Bacon & Chicken

Prep Time: 10 minutes
Cook Time: 8 hours
Total Time: 8 hours 10 minutes
Yield: 6 servings
Serving Size: 1 plate

Bacon obviously makes just about everything better, and chicken is no exception. Chicken - because it's low in fat - can often get a bit dry, especially when you put it in a slow cooker. Adding the bacon to the recipe allows the chicken to stay moist and also allows you to eat more bacon. Win-Win.

INGREDIENTS
- 5 chicken breasts
- 10 slices of bacon
- 2 Tablespoons *(9 g)* thyme *(dried)*
- 1 Tablespoon *(3 g)* oregano *(dried)*
- 1 Tablespoon *(3 g)* rosemary *(dried)*
- 5 Tablespoons *(75 ml)* olive oil *(2 Tbsp (30 ml) for the slow cooker and 3 Tbsp (45 ml) after cooking)*
- 1 Tablespoon *(15 g)* salt

INSTRUCTIONS
1. Place all the ingredients into a slow cooker and mix together.
2. Cook on the low temperature setting for 8 hours.
3. Shred the meat and mix with 3 Tablespoons of olive oil.

SUBSTITUTIONS
- Italian seasoning can be used instead of the thyme, oregano, and rosemary.

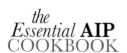

Spinach Basil Chicken Meatballs with Plum Balsamic Sauce

Prep Time: 10 minutes
Cook Time: 15 minutes
Total Time: 25 minutes
Yield: 2 servings
Serving Size: 10-12 meatballs

These are great as an appetizer or as an entree, and the plum balsamic sauce goes really well with the meatballs. If you can't find any plums, don't worry as these also taste great without the sauce!

INGREDIENTS

For the Meatballs:
• 2 chicken breasts *(approx. 1 lb or 454 g)*
• 1/4 lb *(115 g)* spinach
• 2 teaspoons *(10 g)* salt
• 10 basil leaves
• 5 cloves of garlic, peeled
• 3 Tablespoons *(45 ml)* olive oil
• 2 Tablespoons *(30 ml)* olive oil or avocado oil *(to cook in)*

For the Plum Balsamic Sauce:
• 2 plums, pitted
• 1/2 Tablespoon *(7 ml)* balsamic vinegar
• 1/2 Tablespoon *(10.5 g)* of raw honey
• 2 Tablespoons *(30 ml)* water

INSTRUCTIONS

1. Place the chicken breasts, spinach, salt, basil leaves, garlic, and 3 Tablespoons of olive oil into a food processor and process well.
2. Make ping-pong sized meatballs from the meat mixture.
3. Add the 2 Tablespoons olive oil or avocado oil to a frying pan and fry the meatballs for 5 minutes on medium heat *(fry in 2 batches if necessary)*. Turn the meatballs and fry for another 10 minutes. Make sure the meatballs don't get burnt.
4. Meanwhile make the plum balsamic sauce - place the pitted plums, balsamic vinegar, raw honey, and water into a blender and blend well.
5. Pour half the sauce into the frying pan with the meatballs and turn up the heat. Brown the meatballs in the sauce - keep turning the meatballs in the sauce until the sauce is gone and the meatballs are brown.
6. Check the meatballs are fully cooked by cutting into one or using a meat thermometer. Serve with the rest of the plum balsamic sauce.

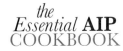

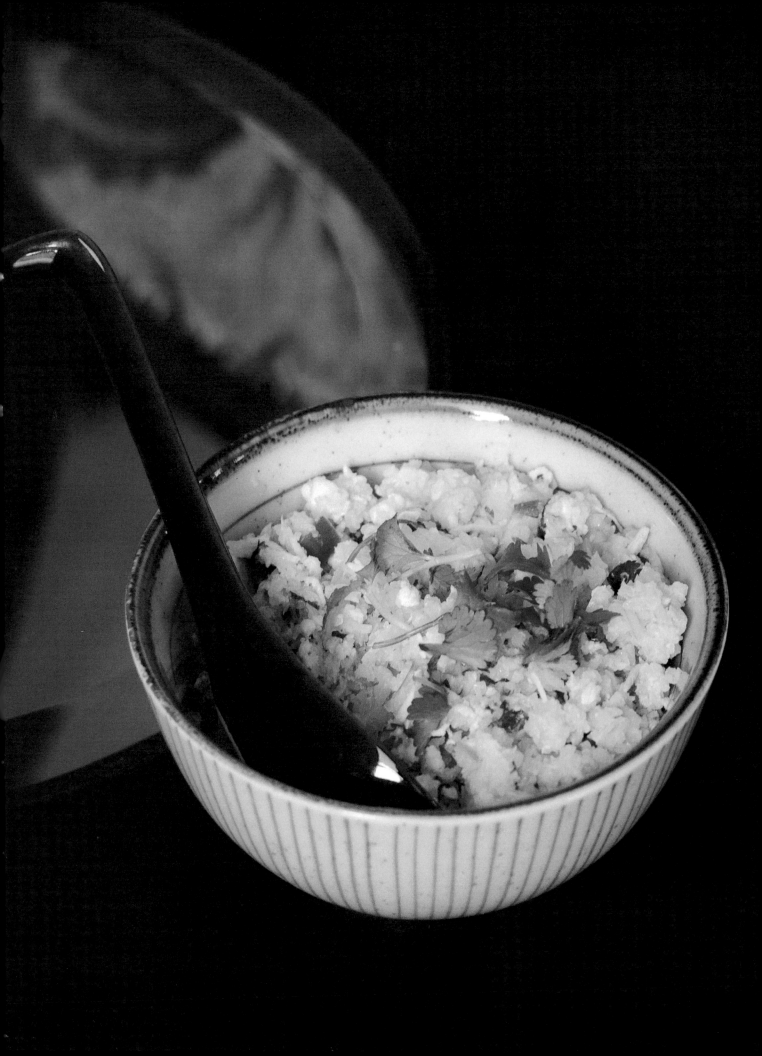

Chicken and "Rice"

Prep Time: 10 minutes
Cook Time: 50 minutes
Total Time: 1 hour
Yield: 4 servings
Serving Size: 1 large bowl

This is another cauliflower rice dish you can try - there are endless variations so feel free to combine some of your favorite vegetables and meats together with cauliflower rice. This recipe is a great way to use leftover meat from a roasted chicken or if you decide to make chicken broth using a whole chicken.

INGREDIENTS

- 1 head of cauliflower
- Meat from a whole roasted chicken *(or use 3-4 cooked chicken breasts)*, shredded
- 1 Tablespoon *(5 g)* freshly grated ginger
- 3 cloves garlic, minced
- 1 Tablespoon *(15 ml)* coconut aminos
- 1/2 cup cilantro, chopped *(for garnish)*
- Coconut oil *(to cook with)*
- Salt *(to taste)*

INSTRUCTIONS

1. If you don't have cooked shredded chicken, poach 3-4 chicken breasts and shred them or use another leftover meat.
2. Break the cauliflower into florets and food process until it forms a rice-like texture *(may need to be done in batches)*.
3. Place the cauliflower into a large pan with coconut oil and cook the cauliflower rice *(may need to be done in 2 pans or in batches)*. Keep the heat on medium and stir regularly.
4. Add in the shredded chicken, ginger, garlic, coconut aminos, cilantro, and salt to taste. Mix together and serve.

SUBSTITUTIONS

- Other leftover meat may be substituted for the chicken.

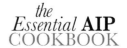

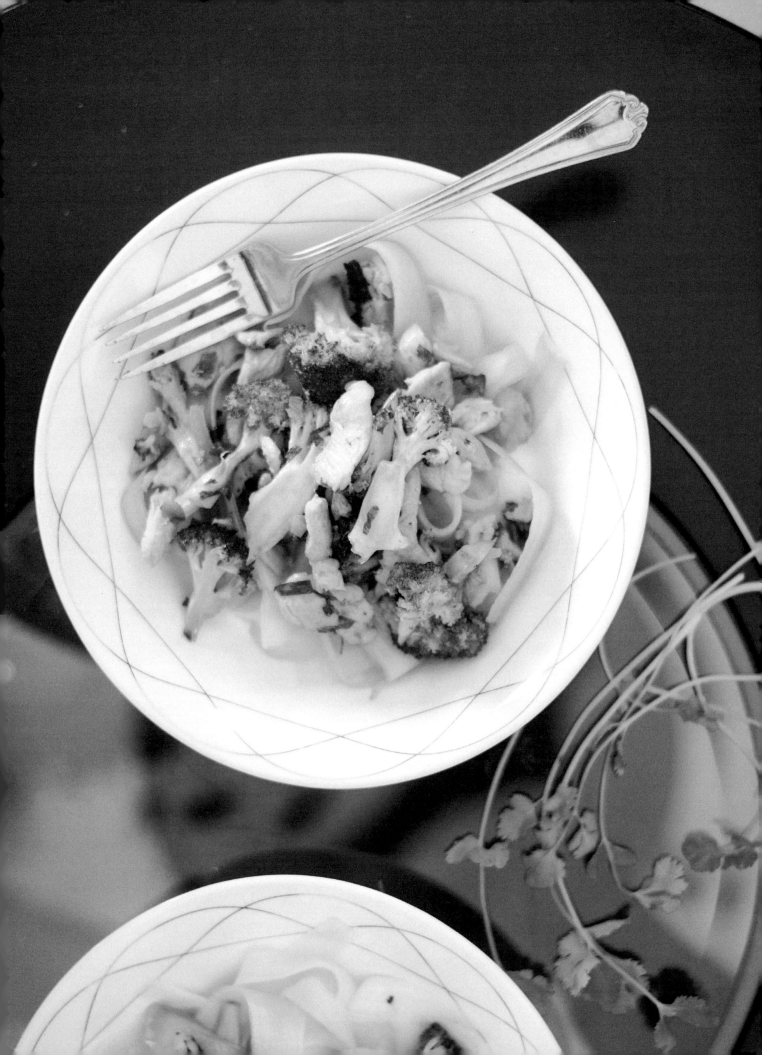

Thai Chicken Pad See Ew

Prep Time: 10 minutes
Cook Time: 15 minutes
Total Time: 25 minutes
Yield: 2 servings
Serving Size: 1 large plate

Pad see ew *(AKA chicken and broccoli stir-fried with flat rice noodles)* is one of my favorite Thai dishes, and you'll find it on the menu at most Thai restaurants. There are lots of different ways to create AIP noodles, but the one I like the most for this dish is to use raw cucumber noodles created using a potato peeler.

INGREDIENTS

- 1 chicken breast *(0.5 lb or 250 g)*, cut into small, thin pieces
- 1/4 cup *(17.5 g)* green onion *(scallions)*, diced
- 1 Tablespoon *(15 ml)* coconut oil *(to cook in)*
- 1 cup *(115 g)* broccoli florets, broken into small florets
- 1 teaspoon *(1.7 g)* freshly grated ginger
- 1 Tablespoon *(15 ml)* coconut aminos
- 2 cloves garlic, minced
- 1 Tablespoon *(15 g)* cilantro, finely chopped
- Salt *(to taste)*
- 1 cucumber, peeled into long noodles using a potato peeler

INSTRUCTIONS

1. Add 1 Tablespoon of coconut oil into a large pan, and saute the chicken breast and green onions in it.

2. Add in the broccoli, ginger, and coconut aminos. Place a lid over the pan and let the broccoli cook on medium heat until it's tender to your liking *(approx. 5-10 minutes)*. Stir regularly.

3. Meanwhile, peel the cucumber and then create the cucumber noodles by using a potato peeler to peel the cucumber into long, wide strands. Divide the cucumber noodles between two plates.

4. Add to the saucepan the minced garlic, cilantro, and salt to taste. Mix and serve on top of the cucumber noodles.

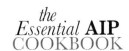

Chapter 3B:
Beef

Beets "No-Tomato" Chili

Prep Time: 15 minutes
Cook Time: 1 hour
Total Time: 1 hour 15 minutes
Yield: 2 servings
Serving Size: 1 plate

It's tough not being able to use tomatoes to flavor dishes on the autoimmune protocol. However, beets are a good substitute - they have a similar color and a slightly milder sweet taste. Give this beets chili a try - I think you'll be surprised at how good it is.

INGREDIENTS

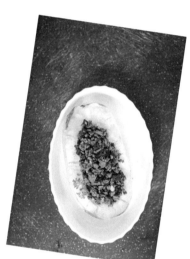

- 1 lb *(454 g)* ground beef
- 1/2 large onion, chopped
- 2 small beets *(approx. 164 g)*, peeled and diced
- 2 cups *(480 ml)* chicken broth or water
- 10 basil leaves, diced
- 4 cloves garlic, minced
- 1/4 cup *(15 g)* fresh parsley, chopped *(optional)*
- Salt *(to taste)*
- Coconut oil *(to cook with)*

INSTRUCTIONS

1. Place 2 Tablespoons of coconut oil into a pan and saute the chopped onion until it turns translucent. Then add in the ground beef and keep sauteing it.
2. Once the beef is cooked, add in the chopped beets to the pan.
3. Add the chicken broth or water to the pan, place a lid on the pan, and simmer on a low heat for 30 minutes. Check on the pan regularly to stir and to make sure it doesn't burn. Add more water if necessary.
4. Once the beets are softened, add the basil, garlic, parsley, and salt to taste.
5. Mix together and serve with Baked Spaghetti Squash *(see Page 132 for recipe)*.

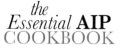

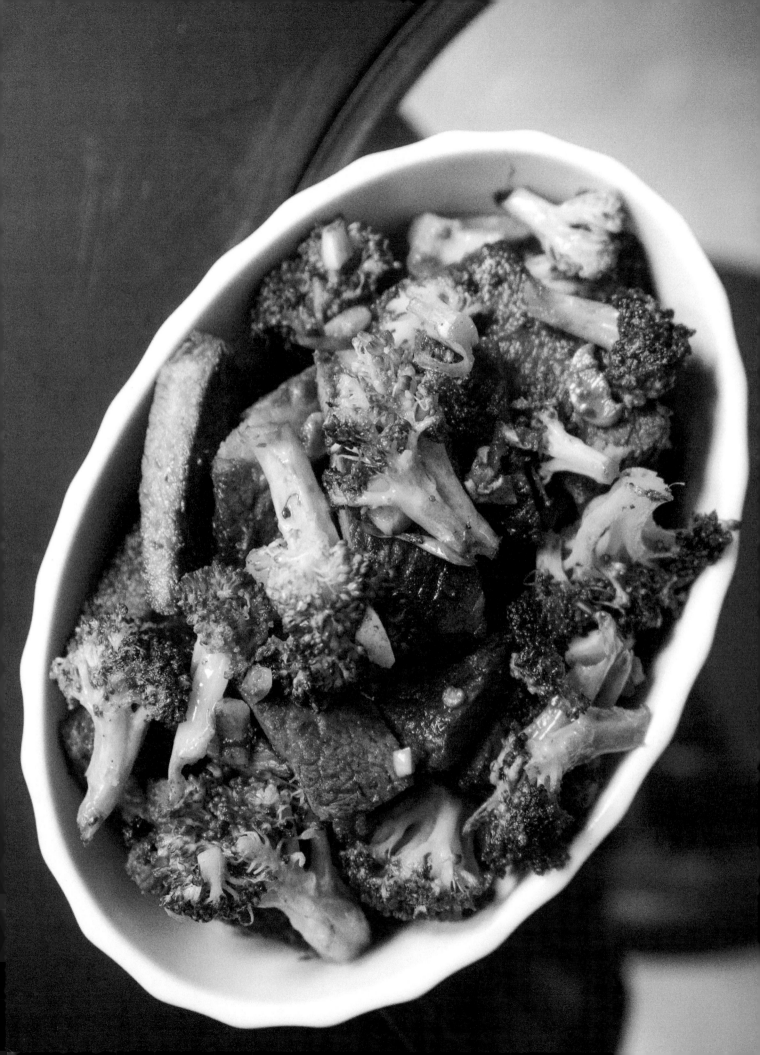

Broccoli Beef

Prep Time: 5 minutes
Cook Time: 15 minutes
Total Time: 20 minutes
Yield: 2 servings
Serving Size: 1 plate

INGREDIENTS

- 2 cups *(182 g)* broccoli florets
- 1/2 lb *(225 g)* beef, sliced thin and precooked *(you can saute it in some coconut oil)*
- 3 cloves garlic, minced *(or use 3/8 teaspoon (0.38 g) garlic powder)*
- 1 teaspoon *(5 g)* freshly grated ginger *(or use ginger powder)*
- 2 Tablespoons *(30 ml)* coconut aminos *(or to taste)*
- Coconut oil *(to cook with)*

INSTRUCTIONS

1. Place 2 Tablespoons of coconut oil into a skillet or saucepan on medium heat. Add the broccoli florets into the skillet.

2. When the broccoli softens to the amount you want *(I like it soft, but some people like it crunchier)*, add in the beef slices.

3. Saute for 2 minutes and then add in the garlic, ginger, and coconut aminos.

4. Serve immediately.

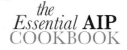

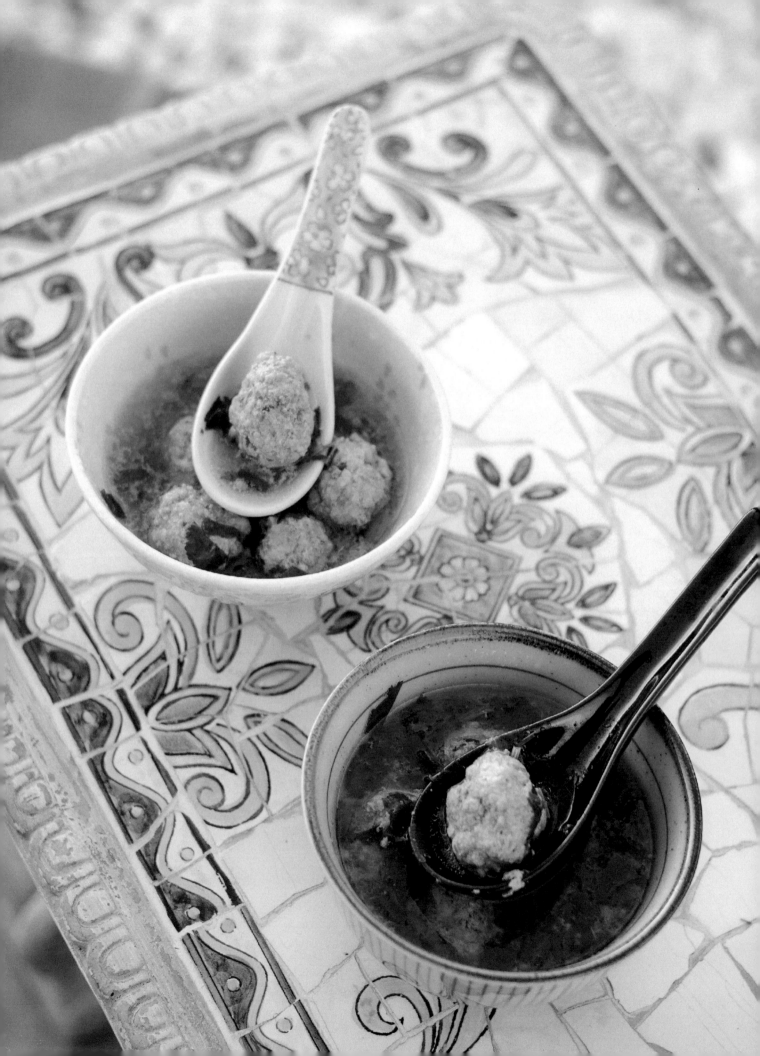

Chinese Meatball Soup

Prep Time: 15 minutes
Cook Time: 15 minutes
Total Time: 30 minutes
Yield: 2 servings
Serving Size: 1 large bowl

INGREDIENTS

- 4 cups *(1 l)* chicken broth or bone broth *(see Page 183 for recipe)*
- 1 teaspoon *(1.7 g)* fresh ginger, grated
- 1/2 lb *(225 g)* ground meat of your choice *(can also be a mix of different ones - I used 1/4 lb of pork with 1/4 lb of beef)*
- 1/4 cup *(15 g)* parsley, chopped
- 5 cloves garlic, minced
- 2 Tablespoons *(4 g)* thyme, fresh *(or 2 teaspoons (2 g) dried thyme)*
- 1/2 Tablespoon *(7.5 g)* salt *(or to taste)*
- 1/4 cup *(15 g)* cilantro, chopped

INSTRUCTIONS

1. Pour the broth into a large pot and set it on a low heat to start simmering. Add in the grated ginger.
2. Meanwhile, in a bowl, mix together the ground meat, parsley, garlic, thyme, and salt.
3. Form approximately 20 meatballs *(just a bit smaller than golf-balls)* with your hands and carefully place into the large pot of broth.
4. Boil for 10-15 minutes *(you can cut one in half to check it's done or use a meat thermometer)*.
5. Add in the cilantro *(and additional salt to taste)*.

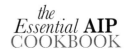

Filet Mignon with Mushroom Sauce

Prep Time: 30 minutes
Cook Time: 30 minutes
Total Time: 1 hour
Yield: 2 servings
Serving Size: 1 filet mignon

INGREDIENTS

- 2 6-oz *(340 g)* filet mignon
- 3 large button mushrooms
- 1 Tablespoon *(10 g)* onions, chopped
- 1 teaspoon *(3 g)* garlic powder
- 1/2 teaspoon *(2.5 g)* salt
- 2 Tablespoons *(30 ml)* olive oil
- Extra salt and olive oil *(for cooking the filet)*

INSTRUCTIONS

1. Preheat oven to 400 F *(200 C)*.
2. Make the sauce by blending the mushrooms, onions, garlic, salt, and olive oil together until pureed.
3. Heat the sauce in a pan for 10 minutes on medium heat.
4. Meanwhile, lightly salt the filet mignons and pan sear them in 2 Tablespoons of olive oil. Finish cooking the filet mignons to the level of doneness you enjoy in the oven *(or in the pan if you prefer)*.
5. Serve with the mushroom sauce.

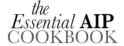

Korean BBQ Beef

Prep Time: 10 minutes
Cook Time: 20 minutes
Total Time: 30 minutes
Yield: 4 servings
Serving Size: 2-3 pieces of beef

INGREDIENTS

- 1-1.5 lb *(454 g - 680 g)* of boneless *(or bone-in)* Korean short ribs *(or use thin strips of beef)*
- 1 apple, peeled and cored
- 1/4 cup *(60 ml)* coconut aminos
- 2 Tablespoons *(30 ml)* avocado oil
- 1 Tablespoon *(15 ml)* apple cider vinegar
- 1/2 teaspoon *(2 g)* garlic powder
- 1 teaspoon *(2 g)* ginger powder
- 1 head of romaine lettuce *(approx. 8 leaves)*

INSTRUCTIONS

1. Fire up the grill to a high temperature.
2. Make the marinade for the beef by placing the apple, coconut aminos, avocado oil, vinegar, garlic powder, and ginger powder into a blender and blend well.
3. Place the strips of beef into the marinade.
4. Grill the beef strips *(or pan-fry them in some avocado oil if preferred).* It only needs a few minutes on each side.
5. Serve with lettuce leaves.

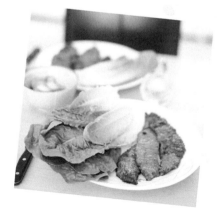

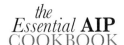

Steak Medallions with Ginger Asparagus Mushroom Saute

Prep Time: 10 minutes
Cook Time: 15 minutes
Total Time: 25 minutes
Yield: 2 servings
Serving Size: 1 plate

This is a whole meal that you can prepare from scratch in under 30 minutes. If you don't have asparagus or mushrooms, then choose some other vegetables.

INGREDIENTS

- 2 beef medallions *(approx. 1/2-3/4 lb or 500-750 g)*
- 6 asparagus shoots, chopped into small slices
- 2 button mushrooms, chopped
- 1/4 onion, chopped
- 1/4 cup *(small handful)* parsley, finely chopped
- 1/2 Tablespoon *(7 g)* fresh ginger, chopped
- Coconut oil *(for frying)*
- Salt *(to taste)*

INSTRUCTIONS

1. Rub salt over the beef medallions *(you can use a beef steak of your choice)*.
2. Place 1 Tablespoon of coconut oil into a frying pan and pan-fry the beef medallions. Alternatively, you can grill the beef. In the frying pan, it only takes 2 minutes on each side for a medium rare level. Cook for longer if you prefer your steak medium or well done.
3. Sit the beef on a plate as some of the liquid will drain out.
4. Meanwhile, in a frying pan, place 1 Tablespoon of coconut oil and add in the chopped onions. Pan-fry the onions until they're translucent. Then add in the asparagus and mushrooms. Saute until the vegetables are soft. Then add in the chopped parsley and ginger. Saute for a few extra minutes and serve with the beef on a new plate.

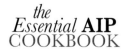

Marinated Grilled Flank Steak

Prep Time: 8 hours *(for marinating)*
Cook Time: 30 minutes
Total Time: 8 hours 30 minutes
Yield: 6 servings
Serving Size: 8-12 oz steak

Flank steak is one of our favorite cuts of beef, but if you're not careful, it can get a bit tough and chewy. A good marinade helps with this, but if you're in a hurry, this dish still tastes great with just 1 hour of marinating.

Enjoy with some Garlic Lemon Broccolini Saute *(see Page 140 for recipe)* as a side dish.

INGREDIENTS

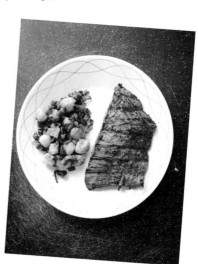

- 3 lbs *(1361 g)* flank steak
- 1 cup *(240 ml)* olive oil
- 2/3 cup *(160 ml)* coconut aminos
- 1/2 cup *(120 ml)* apple cider vinegar
- Juice from 1 lemon
- 6 cloves garlic, minced
- 1 Tablespoon *(5 g)* grated ginger *(or ginger powder)*
- 1 Tablespoon *(7 g)* onion powder
- 1 Tablespoon *(10 g)* garlic powder
- 1 Tablespoon *(15 g)* salt
- 2 teaspoons *(2 g)* dried thyme

INSTRUCTIONS

1. Cut the flank steak into manageable pieces if it's not already cut so.
2. Create the marinade by mixing all ingredients *(except the steak)* in a small bowl.
3. Place each piece of steak into a Ziploc bag and divide the marinade equally among the bags.
4. Seal the bags and marinate the steak overnight.
5. When ready, grill each steak by placing on a hot grill or skillet. Try to turn the steaks as little as possible. You can use a meat thermometer to get the steak to the level of rareness you desire. *(We found 3-4 minutes on each side on a hot 500-600 F grill with the lid down worked well.)*

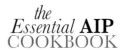

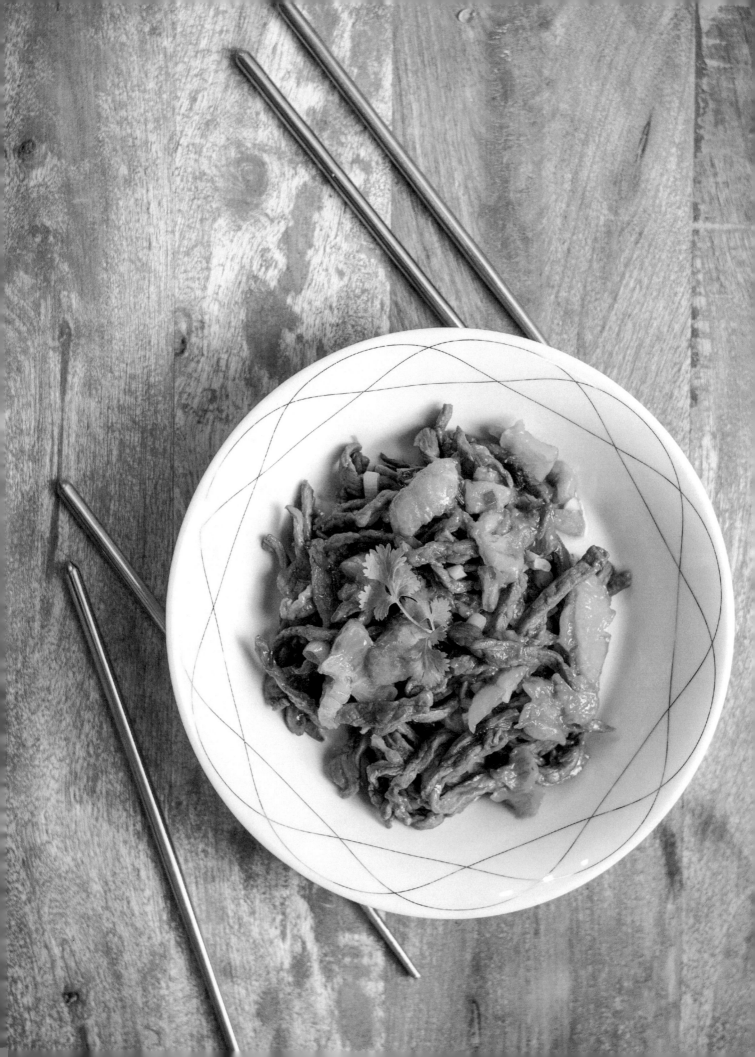

Orange Beef Stir-Fry

Prep Time: 15 minutes
Cook Time: 15 minutes
Total Time: 30 minutes
Yield: 2 servings
Serving Size: 1 plate

Orange chicken is a popular dish in the US, but did you know that orange beef is also delicious? Try this dish with some Cauliflower White "Rice" *(see Page 133 for recipe)* for a Chinese-style AIP dinner. This dish is different to the Orange Chicken Stir-Fry *(see Page 66 for recipe)* as it uses whole pieces of orange rather than creating an orange sauce.

INGREDIENTS
- 1/2 lb *(225 g)* beef round, sliced into thin slices *(1-inch in length)*
- 2 Tablespoons *(8.75 g)* green onions *(scallions)*, chopped
- 2 small oranges, chopped
- 2 cloves garlic, minced
- 1 teaspoon *(1.7 g)* freshly grated ginger *(optional)*
- 2 Tablespoons *(30 ml)* coconut aminos
- 1 Tablespoon *(15 ml)* coconut oil or avocado oil *(to cook in)*
- 1 Tablespoon *(2 g)* cilantro, chopped *(for garnish)*
- Salt *(to taste)*

INSTRUCTIONS
1. Place the coconut or avocado oil into a frying pan. Add in the scallions and then the beef slices and stir-fry on high heat until most of the beef has turned brown.
2. Add in the oranges, garlic, ginger, coconut aminos and saute on high for 2-3 minutes more until the beef is fully cooked.
3. Add salt to taste, garnish with cilantro, and serve.

SUBSTITUTIONS
- 1/4 onion *(chopped)* can be used instead of the scallions.
- Chicken can be used instead of beef.

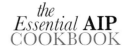
the
Essential **AIP**
COOKBOOK

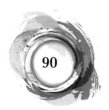

Asian Garlic Beef Noodles

Prep Time: 10 minutes
Cook Time: 20 minutes
Total Time: 30 minutes
Yield: 2 servings
Serving Size: 1 plate

It can be tough giving up pasta and noodles when you're on AIP, but there are many ways to replace them. Zucchini and cucumbers can be sliced into noodles *(you can use a peeler or a spiralizer)*. And shirataki noodles are another easy option.

INGREDIENTS

- 1/2 onion, sliced
- 10 oz *(300 g)* beef, cubed or sliced
- 2 Tablespoons *(30 ml)* avocado oil *(or coconut oil)*
- 2 Tablespoons *(30 ml)* coconut aminos
- 10 cloves garlic, diced
- 1 large chunk of fresh ginger, diced
- 2 Tablespoons *(3.75 g)* cilantro, chopped *(for garnish)*
- 1 zucchini, shredded *(or use a pack of shirataki noodles)*

INSTRUCTIONS

1. Saute the onion slices in the avocado oil.

2. Add in the beef cubes or slices.

3. Add in the coconut aminos.

4. Cook until the beef is tender *(place a lid on the pan to cook it if it needs longer)*.

5. Add in the diced garlic and ginger. Cook for 5 minutes longer.

6. Divide the shredded zucchini or the shirataki noodles between 2 plates. Top with the beef saute.

7. Garnish with the chopped cilantro and serve.

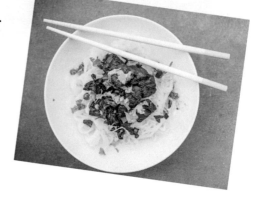

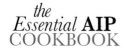

Peach and Steak Salad

Prep Time: 10 minutes
Cook Time: 20 minutes *(to cook the steak)*
Total Time: 30 minutes
Yield: 2 servings
Serving Size: 1 bowl

Many people who start AIP find salads to be one of the easiest foods to make on a daily basis. So if you have some beef left over from another dish, then chop it up and toss it with some greens and a bit of fruit to make a delicious salad.

INGREDIENTS

- 2 peaches
- 1 head of romaine lettuce
- Handful of baby kale leaves
- 2 6-oz *(170 g)* steaks, grilled or pan-fried *(or use leftover Pressure Cooker Beef Short Ribs (recipe on Page 92), Korean BBQ Beef (recipe on Page 85))*
- 3 Tablespoons *(45 ml)* olive oil
- 1 Tablespoon *(15 ml)* balsamic vinegar

INSTRUCTIONS

1. Dice the peaches and the cooked steaks.
2. Toss the peach, steak, romaine lettuce, and kale leaves with the olive oil and balsamic vinegar.

SUBSTITUTIONS

- Nectarines, apricots, or pears can be used instead of peaches.
- Other salad greens can be used instead of romaine lettuce and baby kale leaves.

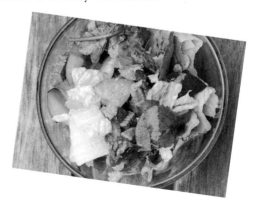

Pressure Cooker Beef Short Ribs

Prep Time: 10 minutes
Cook Time: 1 hour
Total Time: 1 hour 10 minutes
Yield: 4 servings
Serving Size: 1 plate

If you don't have a pressure cooker, you can use a slow cooker instead to make this. You can use leftovers to make the Sweet Potato Breakfast Hash *(see Page 36 for recipe)*, the Orange Beef Stir-Fry *(see Page 88 for recipe)*, or as a replacement for bacon in the Easy Bacon Brussels Sprouts recipe *(see Page 137 for recipe)*.

INGREDIENTS
- 2 lbs *(1 kg)* boneless beef short ribs *(or 4 lbs bone-in beef short ribs)*
- 1 onion, diced
- 1 carrot, diced
- 1 cup *(240 ml)* water
- 3 Tablespoons *(45 ml)* coconut aminos
- 1 Tablespoon *(15 g)* salt

INSTRUCTIONS
1. Place all the ingredients into a pressure cooker.
2. Press the Meat/Stew button *(normal pressure)* and then set the timer for 45 minutes. *(The pressure cooker takes a few minutes of prep to get ready and then a few minutes to bring the pressure down, so the total cook time is closer to 1 hour.)*

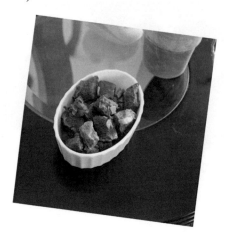

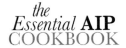

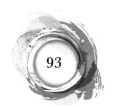

Slow Cooker Beef Stew

Prep Time: 10 minutes
Cook Time: 8 hours
Total Time: 8 hours, 10 minutes
Yield: 6 servings
Serving Size: 1 bowl

The reason I have so many slow cooker recipes in this cookbook is because they make your life and diet so much easier. I absolutely love putting something in at night, having it ready the next day to eat, and then having leftovers that we can eat for several days.

INGREDIENTS

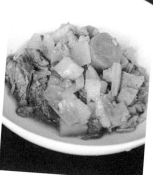

- 2.5 lbs *(1.1 kg)* beef *(stew meat or short ribs meat)*
- 4 carrots
- 2 white parsnips
- 2 sweet potatoes
- 1 small onion
- 4 celery sticks
- 2 cloves garlic, minced
- 2 cups *(480 ml)* broth *(e.g., bone broth or water)*
- 2 teaspoons *(10 g)* salt
- 1 teaspoon *(3 g)* garlic powder
- 1 teaspoon *(2 g)* onion powder

INSTRUCTIONS

1. Chop up the beef into 1-inch *(2.5 cm)* cubes if you're not using stew meat.

2. Pour the broth into the bottom of the slow cooker.

3. Place the meat into the slow cooker.

4. Season the meat in the slow cooker with salt, garlic powder, onion powder, and minced garlic.

5. Chop up the vegetables into rough 1-inch *(2.5 cm)* cubes and place on top of the meat in the slow cooker.

6. Place the lid on the slow cooker and cook on the low temperature setting for 8 hours.

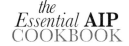

the Essential **AIP**
COOKBOOK

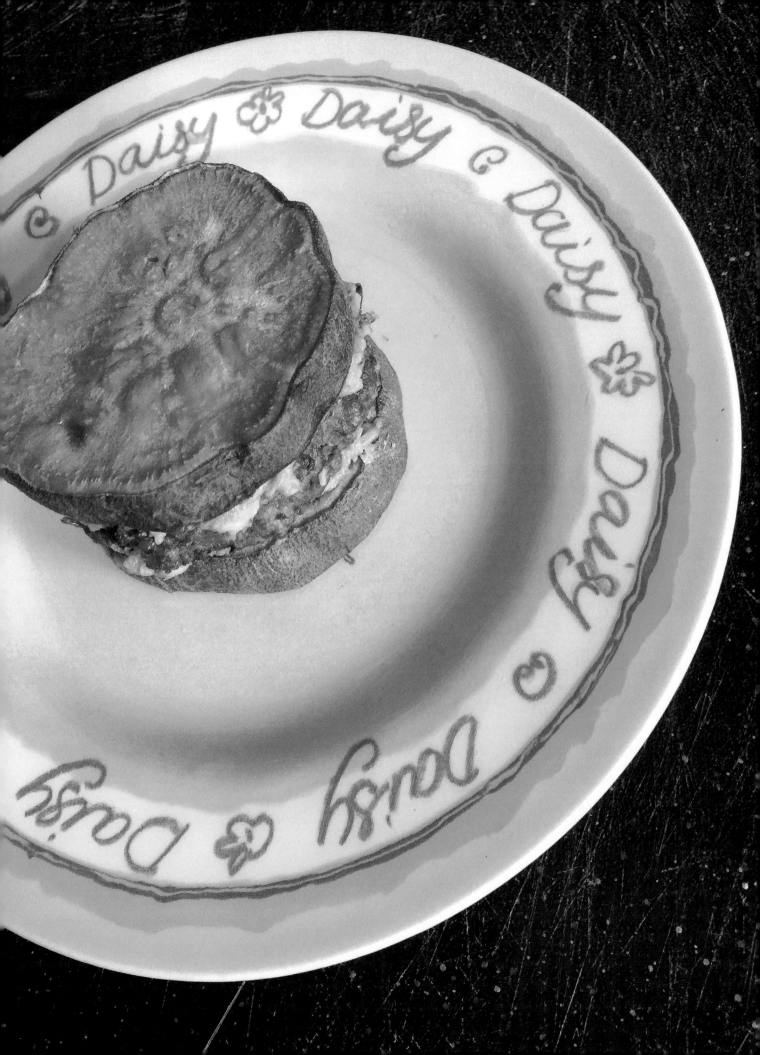

Sweet Potato Guacamole Burger

Prep Time: 10 minutes
Cook Time: 30 minutes
Total Time: 40 minutes
Yield: 2 servings
Serving Size: 2 burgers

These burgers are surprisingly easy to make and super delicious. While store-bought guacamole typically contains nightshades like tomatoes and peppers, you can easily make your own AIP guacamole following the recipe below.

Enjoy with some Parsnip Fries *(see Page 144 for recipe)* for a burger and fries dinner.

INGREDIENTS

- 4 small beef patties *(approx. 1/2 lb or 225 g minced beef)*
- 1 avocado, mashed
- 1/2 lime, juiced
- 1 teaspoon *(3 g)* garlic powder
- 1 Tablespoon *(3.75 g)* cilantro, chopped
- Salt *(to taste)*
- 8 large slices of sweet potato *(1/2-inch thick)*
- Coconut oil to cook with

INSTRUCTIONS

1. Preheat oven to 350 F *(175 C)*.
2. Place the sweet potato slices on a baking tray and bake for 30 minutes until slightly tender.
3. Meanwhile, cook the burger patties, either in a skillet with a bit of coconut oil or on a grill. Once the burgers are cooked through, place to the side.
4. Make the guacamole using the mashed avocado, lime juice, garlic powder, cilantro, and salt.
5. Put together the 4 burgers and serve.

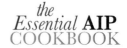

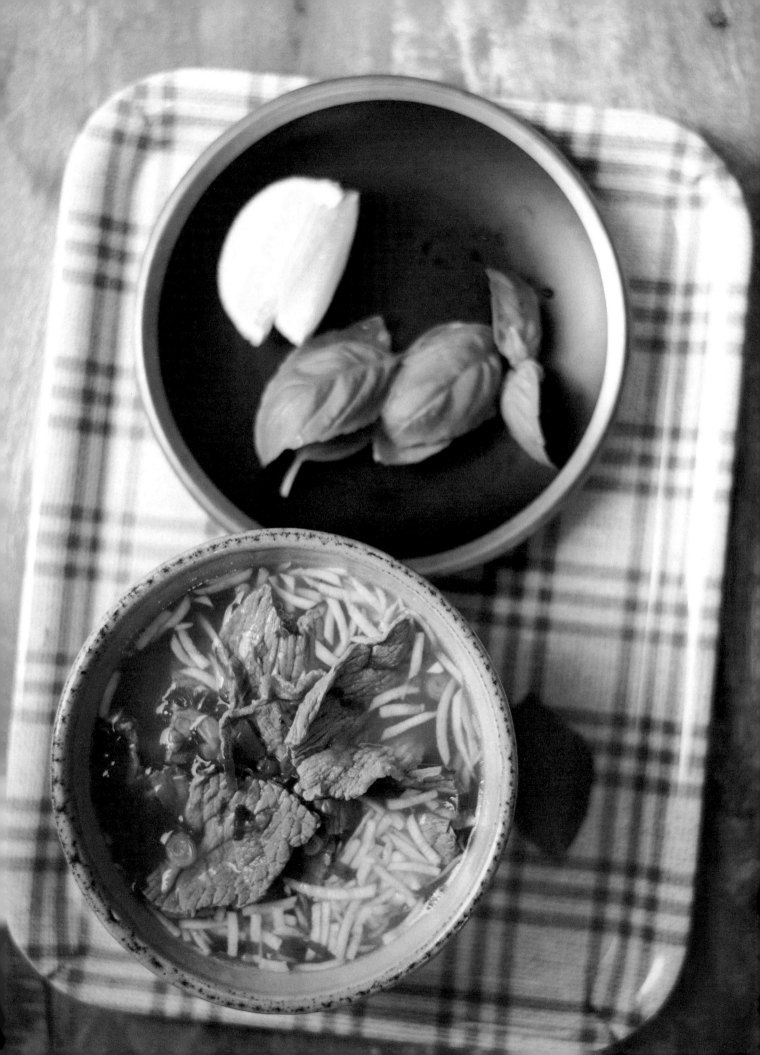

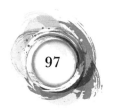

Vietnamese Beef Pho

Prep Time: 15 minutes
Cook Time: 10 minutes
Total Time: 25 minutes
Yield: 2 servings
Serving Size: 1 bowl

INGREDIENTS

- 3 cups *(720 ml)* bone broth *(or chicken broth) (see Page 183 for recipe)*
- 1/2 lb *(225 g)* beef round, sliced very thin
- 1 teaspoon *(1.7 g)* ginger, grated *(or use 1/2 teaspoon (0.5 g) ginger powder)*
- 1/2 teaspoon *(1 g)* cinnamon powder
- 2 zucchinis, shredded *(or 2 packs of shirataki noodles)*
- 2 green onions *(scallions)*, chopped
- 1/4 cup *(15 g)* cilantro, finely diced
- Salt *(to taste)*
- 10 basil leaves
- 1/2 lime, cut into 4 wedges

INSTRUCTIONS

1. Slice the beef round very thinly against the grain *(tip: freeze the beef for 20-30 minutes before cutting to get thinner slices)*.

2. Heat up the broth.

3. When the broth starts boiling, add in the freshly grated ginger, cinnamon powder, and salt to taste.

4. Add in the beef slices slowly, making sure they don't all clump together.

5. Then add in the zucchini noodles, the green onions, and the cilantro.

6. Cook for 1 minute until the beef slices are done.

7. Serve with the basil leaves and lime wedges.

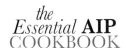

Chapter 3C:

Pork

Bacon Acorn Squash Mash

Prep Time: 10 minutes
Cook Time: 50 minutes
Total Time: 1 hour
Yield: 2 servings
Serving Size: 1 large bowl

This recipe is named for the Acorn Squash, but it's really the bacon and collard greens that make all the difference.

INGREDIENTS

- 1 lb *(454 g)* bacon, uncooked, chopped into small pieces
- 10 ounces *(284 g)* collard greens *(approx. 1 bunch)*, chopped into small pieces
- 2 medium-sized acorn squash
- 1/2 navel orange, peeled and finely chopped
- Pinch of saffron *(optional - crush and soak for 30 minutes in warm water)*

INSTRUCTIONS

1. Halve the acorn squash and remove the seeds. Soften the inside of the squash by baking on a baking tray in the oven for 40 minutes at 400 F *(200 C)* or microwave on high for 3-4 minutes.
2. Cook the bacon pieces in a pot until crispy.
3. Boil the collard greens in a pot of boiling water for 40 minutes until tender. Add to the pot with the bacon.
4. Scoop out the inside of the acorn squash when it's tender and place into the pot with the bacon pieces and the collard greens.
5. Add the orange and saffron *(optional)* to the pot and cook on a low heat. Stir until the acorn squash forms a mash consistency *(5-10 minutes)*. Serve immediately.

SUBSTITUTIONS

• Butternut squash can be used instead of acorn squash.

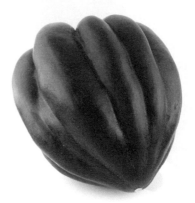

the Essential **AIP**
COOKBOOK

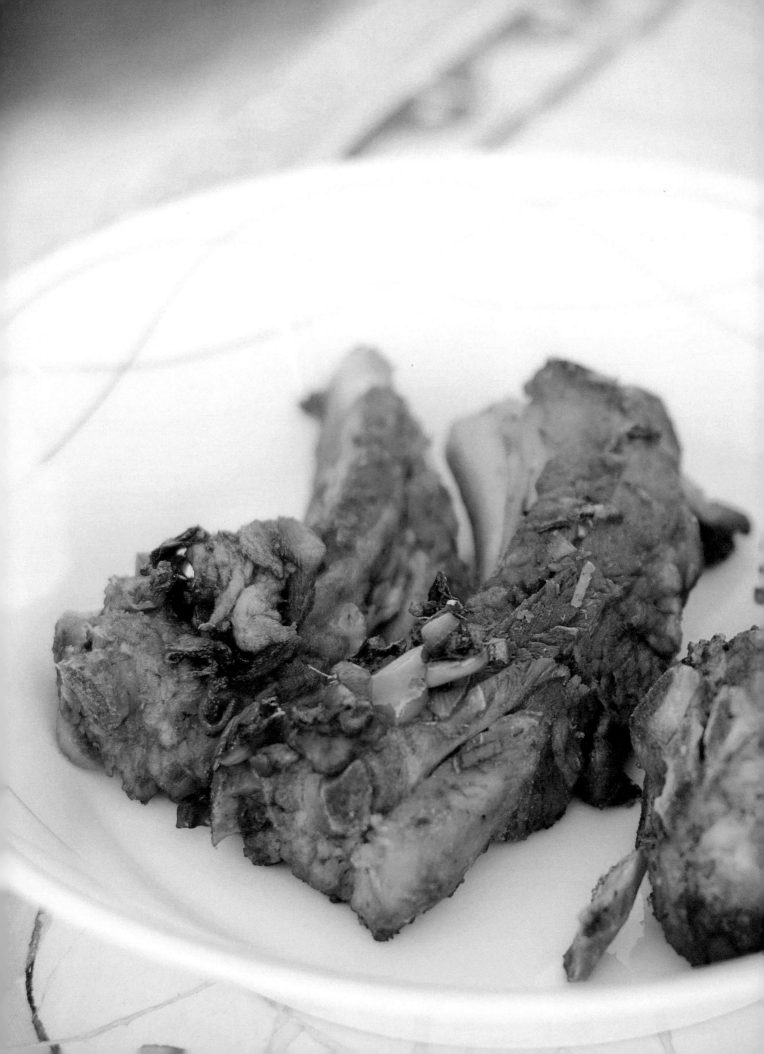

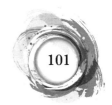

Chinese Pork Spare Ribs

Prep Time: 10 minutes
Cook Time: 1 hour 20 minutes
Total Time: 1 hour 30 minutes
Yield: 4 servings
Serving Size: 1 lb (454 g) of ribs

INGREDIENTS

- 4 lbs *(1.8 kg)* pork spare ribs *(or back ribs)*, chopped into individual ribs
- 1/2 inch *(1.25 cm)* chunk of fresh ginger, sliced into 2 pieces
- 1/2 inch *(1.25 cm)* chunk of fresh ginger, finely diced
- 1/2 cup *(35 g)* scallions *(green onions)*, diced and divided into 2 parts
- 2 Tablespoons *(30 g)* salt *(optional)*
- 6 cloves garlic, minced
- 4 Tablespoons *(60 ml)* coconut aminos
- 4 Tablespoons *(60 ml)* avocado oil

INSTRUCTIONS

1. Place the ribs in a large stockpot filled with water so that the ribs are covered.
2. After the water starts boiling, skim off any foam that forms on the top of the broth *(for prettiness)*.
3. Add the 2 slices of ginger, 1/4 cup of scallions, and 2 Tablespoons of salt to the pot and simmer until the meat is cooked and soft *(approx. 45 minutes)*.
4. Remove the ribs from the pot but keep the broth *(pour it through a sieve to remove all solids)*. The broth *(by itself)* is wonderful to drink or else you can use it as the base for delicious soups.
5. In a small bowl, mix together the diced ginger, rest of the scallions, minced garlic, coconut aminos, and the 2 Tablespoons of avocado oil.
6. Heat up a skillet *(or wok if you have one)* on high heat and add the ribs in batches to it. Divide the mixture so that you will have enough for each batch of ribs. Coat each batch of ribs on both sides with the mixture. Double the mixture if you prefer more sauce on the ribs.
7. Saute the ribs on high heat until they brown and no more liquid remains in the skillet.

SUBSTITUTIONS

- Half an onion, diced, can be used instead of the 1/2 cup scallions.

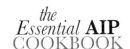

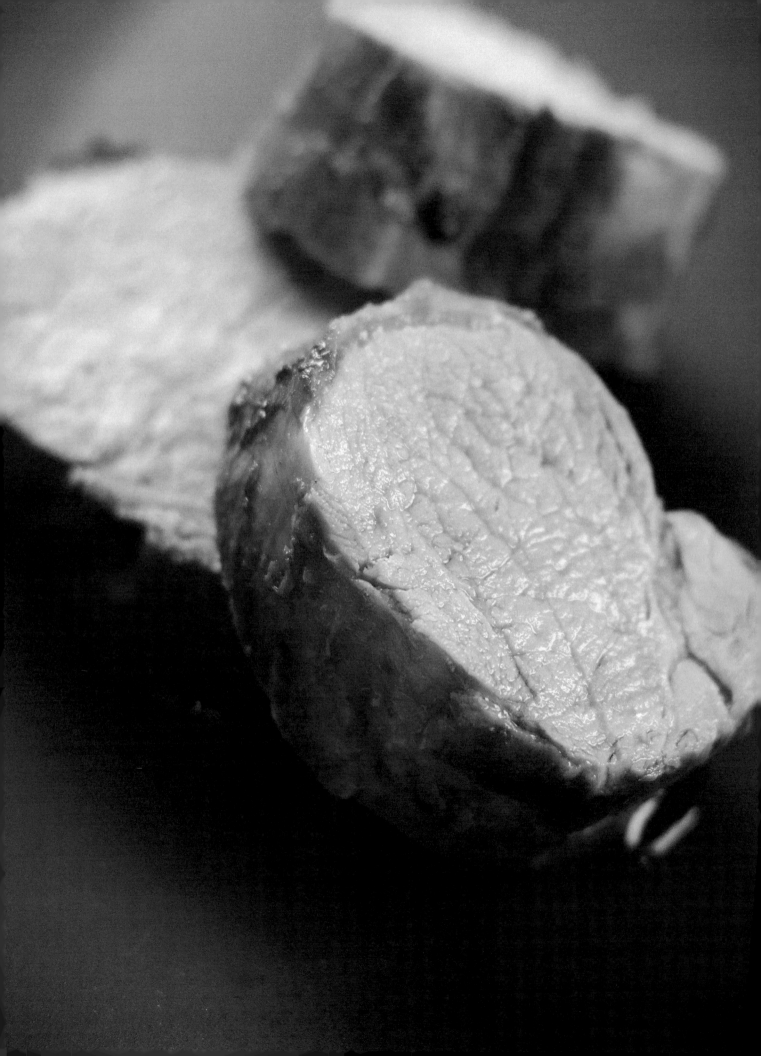

Pan-Fried Pork Tenderloin

Prep Time: 10 minutes
Cook Time: 20 minutes
Total Time: 30 minutes
Yield: 2 servings
Serving Size: 1/2 lb *(225 g)* of pork

INGREDIENTS

- 1 lb *(454 g)* pork tenderloin
- Salt *(to taste)*
- 1 Tablespoon *(15 ml)* coconut oil *(for cooking with)*

Optional peach and basil balsamic sauce:

- 2 peaches, peeled and chopped into pieces
- 4 basil leaves
- 1 teaspoon *(5 ml)* balsamic vinegar
- 2 Tablespoons *(15 ml)* coconut oil
- 1 teaspoon *(7 g)* raw honey *(optional)*

INSTRUCTIONS

1. Cut the 1 lb pork tenderloin in half *(to create 2 equal shorter halves)*.

2. Place the 1 Tablespoon of coconut oil into a frying pan on a medium heat.

3. After the coconut oil melts, place the 2 pork tenderloin pieces into the pan.

4. Leave the pork to cook on its side. Once that side is cooked, turn using tongs to cook the other sides. Keep turning and cooking until the pork looks cooked on all sides.

5. Cook all sides of the pork until the meat thermometer shows an internal temperature of just below 145 F *(63 C)*. The pork will keep on cooking a bit after you take it out of the pan.

6. Let the pork sit for a few minutes and then slice into 1-inch thick slices with a sharp knife.

7. To make the optional sauce, puree the peach pieces, basil, balsamic vinegar, coconut oil, and honey together.

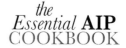

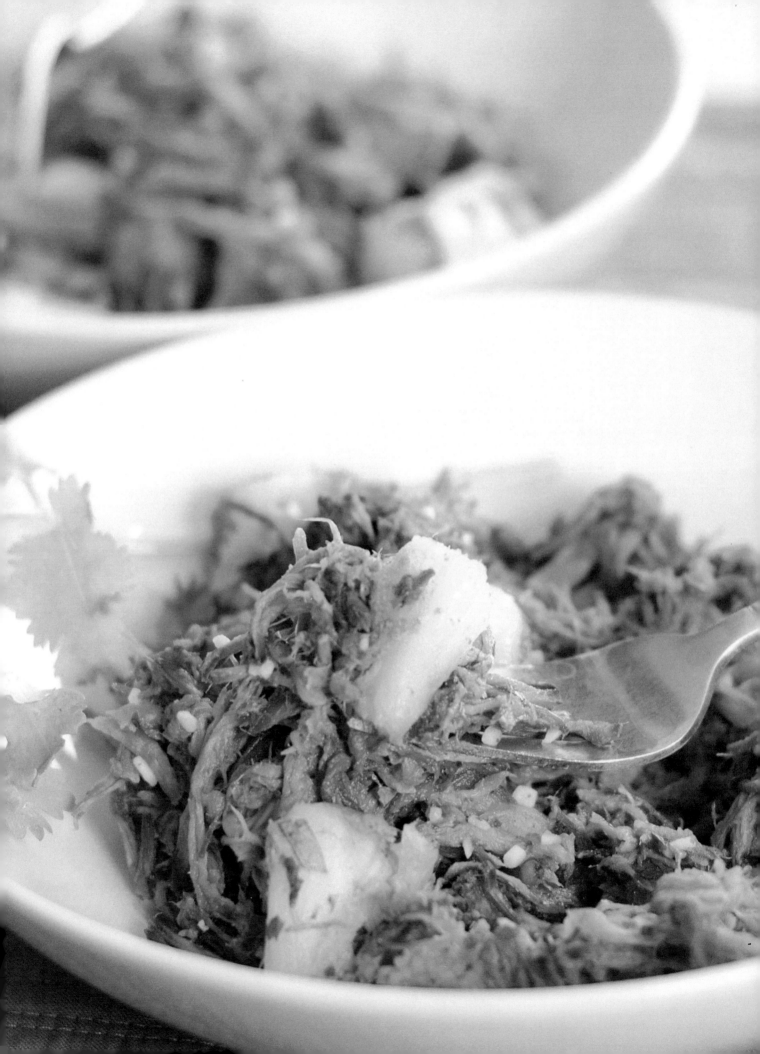

Pineapple Pork

Prep Time: 5 minutes
Cook Time: 10 minutes
Total Time: 15 minutes
Yield: 2 servings
Serving Size: 1 medium bowl

If you've been following us for any length of time *(or if you've seen some of Jeremy's videos)*, then you probably know that this is his absolute favorite recipe. Part of that is because he's lazy and loves how fast this dish can be prepared. Another part of it is because it's just so yummy.

INGREDIENTS

- 2 cups *(490 g)* pineapple chunks *(frozen or fresh)*
- 3 cups *(747 g)* shredded pork *(see Page 108 for recipe)*
- 1 teaspoon *(1.7 g)* freshly grated ginger
- 3 cloves garlic, minced
- 1/4 cup *(15 g)* cilantro, chopped
- Salt *(to taste)*
- 1 Tablespoon *(15 ml)* coconut oil *(to cook in)*

INSTRUCTIONS

1. Melt 1 Tablespoon of coconut oil in a saucepan and add in the pineapple chunks. Cook until the pineapple chunks are softened.
2. Add in the shredded pork and cook for 5 minutes.
3. Add in the ginger, garlic, cilantro, and season with salt to taste.

SUBSTITUTIONS

• Cilantro and ginger can be omitted.
• Garlic powder can be used instead of fresh garlic.

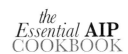

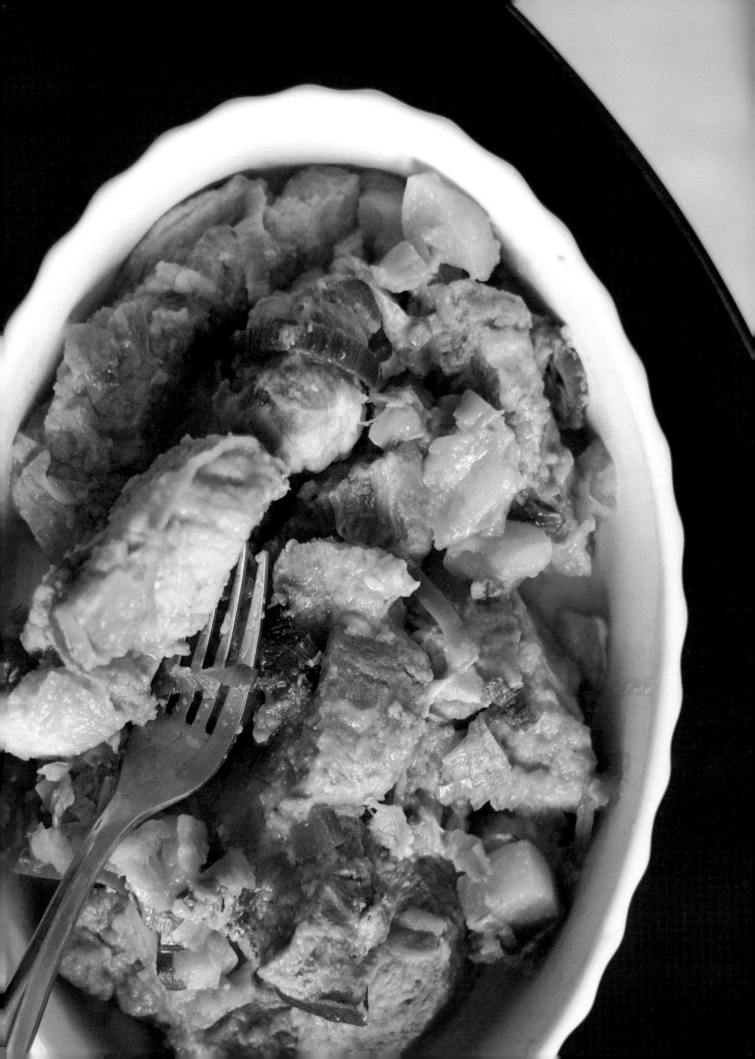

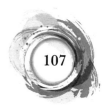

Pressure Cooker Pork and Apple

Prep Time: 10 minutes
Cook Time: 40 minutes
Total Time: 50 minutes
Yield: 2-3 servings
Serving Size: 1 plate

Apple goes so well with pork, and in this recipe, I combined the apple and pork so that the flavors can mix together in the pressure cooker.

While I love cooking with my slow cooker, it is often convenient to use the pressure cooker for cooking dinners if I didn't plan ahead well enough. It's just so much faster at cooking meats and making them super tender.

INGREDIENTS

- 1 apple, peeled and chopped
- 1 lb *(454 g)* pork shoulder
- 1/4 cup *(60 ml)* apple sauce *(or use 1-2 Tablespoons raw honey)*
- 1 Tablespoon *(5 g)* fresh ginger, grated or as 1 large chunk *(or use 1 teaspoon (1 g) ginger powder)*
- 1/4 cup leek *(or onion)*, chopped
- Salt *(to taste)*

INSTRUCTIONS

1. Place all the ingredients into the pressure cooker and set it for 40 minutes on normal pressure.
2. Add more salt or apple sauce to taste and serve hot.

SUBSTITUTIONS

- You can of course make this same dish in the slow cooker instead. Just place into the slow cooker for 6-8 hours on low until the pork is tender.

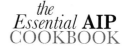

the
Essential **AIP**
COOKBOOK

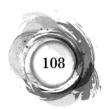
Slow Cooker Shredded Pork

Prep Time: 5 minutes
Cook Time: 8 hours
Total Time: 8 hours 5 minutes
Yield: 4 servings
Serving Size: 1/2 lb *(227 g)* pork

I highly suggest putting your slow cooker to good use!

And you don't have to make anything fancy in them - sometimes just a piece of meat with some salt is all you need. Then you can use that tender cooked meat in a variety of ways to make your meals quickly and easily. For example, this shredded pork can be used in the Pineapple Pork dish *(see Page 104 for recipe)* or as a leftover meat in soups and other sautes.

You can use this same recipe to cook other meats like beef roasts.

INGREDIENTS
- 2 lbs *(908 g)* pork shoulder *(or pork shoulder collar)*
- 1 Tablespoon *(15 g)* salt *(or to taste)*
- 1 Tablespoon *(5 g)* ginger powder or fresh ginger *(optional)*

INSTRUCTIONS
1. Place the pork into the slow cooker *(leave the pork whole - do not cut it up)*.
2. Sprinkle the salt and ginger powder onto the meat.
3. Set the slow cooker for 8 hours on low heat setting.
4. Turn the pork over after 6 hours but do not pull it apart. Shred the pork when serving to prevent drying.
5. Serve by itself or use it to make Pineapple Pork *(see Page 104 for recipe)*.

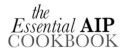

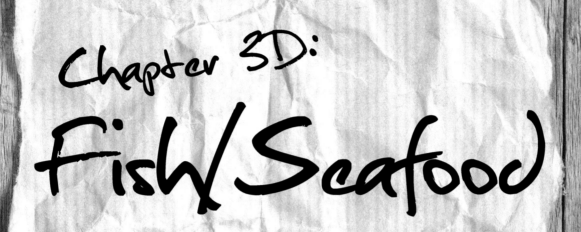

Chapter 5D:
Fish/Seafood

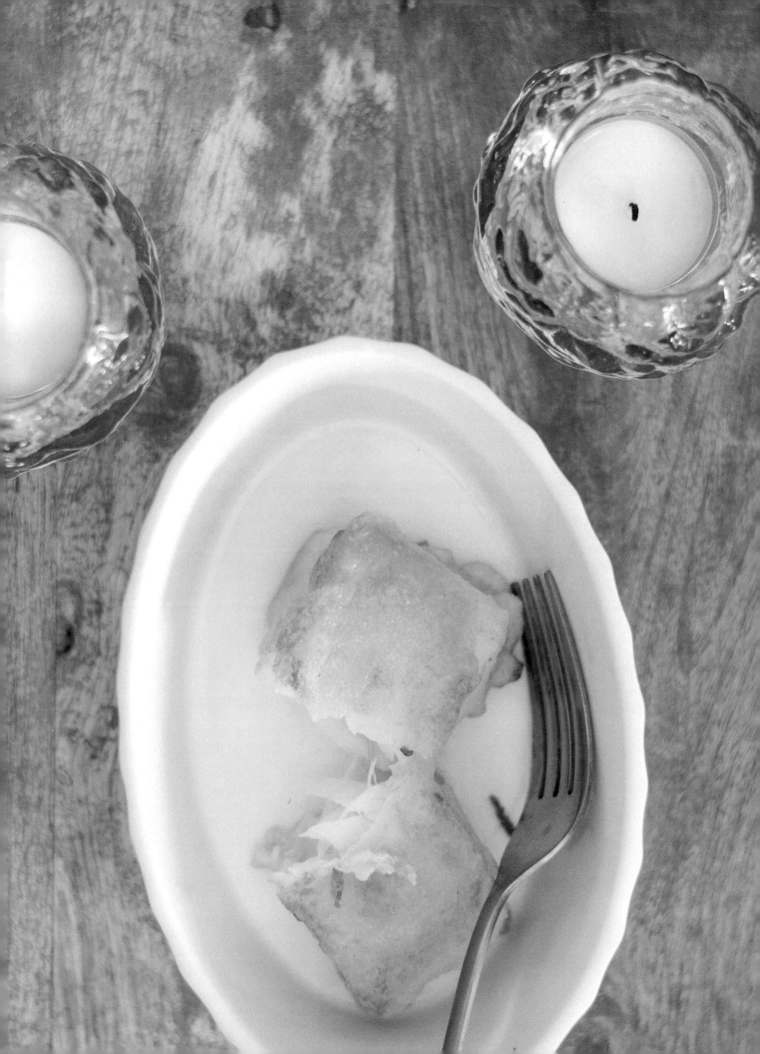

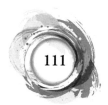

Arrowroot Battered Fish

Prep Time: 10 minutes
Cook Time: 10 minutes
Total Time: 20 minutes
Yield: 1 serving
Serving Size: 1 plate

Arrowroot flour is a really useful flour for AIP cooking - it behaves differently to regular wheat flour, but it is useful for thickening stews and sauces as well as for making thin batters like in this recipe. Of course, it is not necessary to have arrowroot flour for AIP - it's just nice to have around if you want to recreate some "bread"-like foods.

INGREDIENTS

- 1/2 lb *(225 g)* white fish
- Avocado oil *(for frying)*

For the Batter:

- 1/4 cup *(36 g)* arrowroot flour
- 1 Tablespoon *(7 g)* coconut flour
- 1 teaspoon *(3 g)* garlic powder
- Dash of salt
- 2-3 Tablespoons *(30-45 ml)* cold water

INSTRUCTIONS

1. Cut the fish into 2-inch by 1-inch chunks.
2. Make the batter by mixing together all the dry batter ingredients. Add 2 Tablespoons *(30 ml)* of water initially and then slowly add in the third Tablespoon if needed to make the arrowroot flour form a batter.
3. Place 2 Tablespoons *(30 ml)* of avocado oil into a frying pan on medium heat.
4. Coat each chunk of fish with the batter ingredients and quickly place into the avocado oil as the batter comes off easily. Fry for several minutes on each side until the batter turns golden. Check the fish is fully cooked before serving.
5. Serve with some Parsnip Fries *(see Page 144 for recipe)* for a fish and chips dinner.

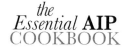

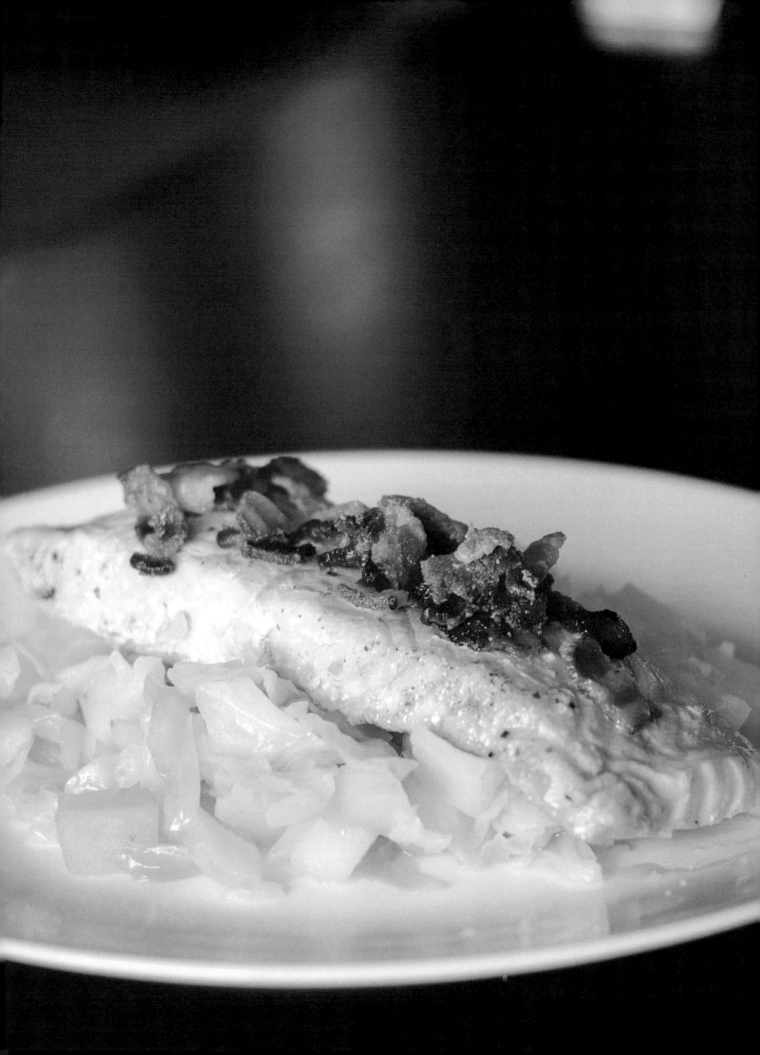

Baked Salmon with Cabbage, Apple, and Fennel

Prep Time: 10 minutes
Cook Time: 30 minutes
Total Time: 40 minutes
Yield: 4 servings
Serving Size: 1 plate

INGREDIENTS

- 4 salmon filets
- 1/2 cup *(120 ml)* olive oil
- 1/2 head of cabbage, chopped into small pieces
- 1 head of fennel, diced *(or use 1 celery heart)*
- 2 apples, peeled and diced
- 1/2 cup *(120 ml)* chicken broth *(or water)*
- 4 Tablespoons *(60 ml)* coconut oil
- 3-4 slices of bacon, chopped into pieces *(optional)*
- Salt *(to taste)*

INSTRUCTIONS

1. Preheat oven to 350 F *(175 C)*.

2. Place each salmon filet onto a piece of aluminum foil or parchment paper with 2 Tablespoons of olive oil and a bit of salt. Wrap up each filet in foil or paper and place in the oven for 30 minutes.

3. While the salmon is baking, place the coconut oil into a large saucepan and add in the cabbage and chicken broth and put the lid on the saucepan. After 10 minutes, add in the fennel, stir and keep the lid on. After another 10 minutes, add in the apples. Stir and season with salt. Cook until the salmon is done.

4. Place the cabbage mixture on a plate, place the salmon on top, then top with bacon pieces.

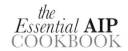

the
Essential **AIP**
COOKBOOK

Boiled Dungeness Crab

Prep Time: 0 minute
Cook Time: 15 minutes
Total Time: 15 minutes
Yield: 2 servings
Serving Size: 1/2 crab

I'm a huge fan of crab meat - it's nutritious and delicious. So, if you can get a whole fresh crab *(often Asian supermarkets or fresh fish markets will sell them)*, then give this recipe a try.

Enjoy with some Chinese Bamboo Salad *(see Page 42 for recipe)* as an appetizer.

INGREDIENTS

- 1 dungeness crab

INSTRUCTIONS

1. Place the crab into a large pot of cold water - use long tongs for live crabs.
2. Bring the pot of cold water to the boil slowly.
3. Boil for 7-8 minutes per lb of crab.

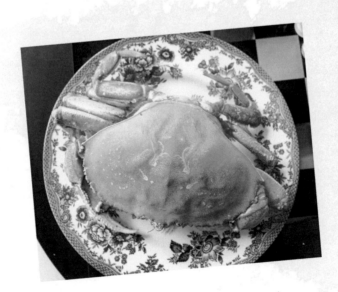

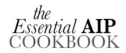

"Breaded" Fish with Garlic Sauce

Prep Time: 10 minutes
Cook Time: 20 minutes
Total Time: 30 minutes
Yield: 4 servings
Serving Size: 1 piece of cod

This coconut breading mixture is easy to make and delicious to eat. And if you don't want to use coconut oil for the sauce, you can use olive oil instead.

Enjoy with a large helping of Creamy Cauliflower Mash *(see Page 135 for recipe)*.

INGREDIENTS
- 4 cod filets *(approx. 0.3 lb or 135 g each) (or use other fish)*
- 1/2 cup *(56 g)* coconut flour
- 2 Tablespoons *(10 g)* shredded coconut
- 3 Tablespoons *(30 g)* garlic powder
- 1 Tablespoon *(7 g)* onion powder
- Salt *(to taste)*
- 2 Tablespoons *(30 ml)* coconut oil
- 3 cloves garlic, minced
- Coconut oil *(for greasing baking tray)*

INSTRUCTIONS
1. Preheat oven to 425 F *(220 C)*.
2. In a large bowl, combine the breading ingredients *(coconut flour, shredded coconut, garlic powder, and onion powder)*. Add in salt and taste the mixture to see how much salt you like.
3. Cover a baking tray with aluminum foil or parchment paper and grease with coconut oil.
4. Dip each fish filet into the breading mixture and cover well. Place the breaded fish onto the baking tray.
5. Bake for 15-20 minutes until the fish flakes easily.
6. While the fish is in the oven, prepare the garlic sauce by melting the coconut oil slightly and adding in the minced garlic.
7. Pour the garlic sauce on top of the breaded fish and serve.

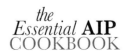

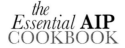

Cucumber Ginger Shrimp

Prep Time: 5 minutes
Cook Time: 10 minutes
Total Time: 15 minutes
Yield: 1 serving
Serving Size: 1 plate

This recipe is super simple and fast! Enjoy it with some slices of Lemon Fried Avocado Slices *(see Page 55 for recipe)* for a filling and quick meal.

INGREDIENTS

- 1 large cucumber, peeled and sliced into 1/2-inch round slices
- 10-15 large shrimp/prawns *(defrosted if frozen)*
- 1 teaspoon *(1.7 g)* fresh ginger, grated
- Salt *(to taste)*
- Coconut oil *(to cook with)*

INSTRUCTIONS

1. Place 1 Tablespoon *(15 ml)* of coconut oil into a frying pan on medium heat.
2. Add in the ginger and the cucumber and saute for 2-3 minutes.
3. Add in the shrimp/prawns and cook until they turn pink and are no longer translucent.
4. Add salt to taste and serve.

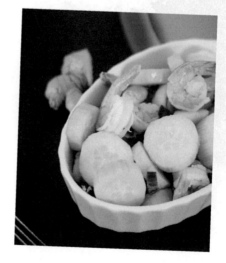

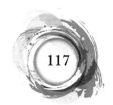

Fish and Leek Saute

Prep Time: 10 minutes
Cook Time: 10 minutes
Total Time: 20 minutes
Yield: 2 servings
Serving Size: 1 plate

Enjoy with a side of Ginger and Garlic Bok Choy Stir-Fry *(see Page 141 for recipe)*.

INGREDIENTS

- 2 fish filets *(approx. 8 oz or 230 g each)*, diced
- 1 leek, chopped
- 1 teaspoon *(1.7 g)* grated ginger
- 1 Tablespoon *(15 ml)* coconut aminos
- Salt *(to taste)*
- 1 Tablespoon *(15 ml)* avocado oil

INSTRUCTIONS

1. Add the avocado oil into a skillet and saute the chopped leek.

2. When the leeks soften, add the diced fish, grated ginger, coconut aminos, and salt to taste.

3. Saute until the fish isn't translucent anymore and is cooked. Serve immediately.

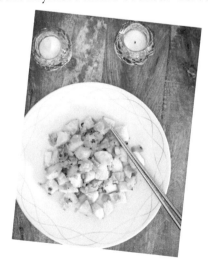

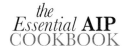

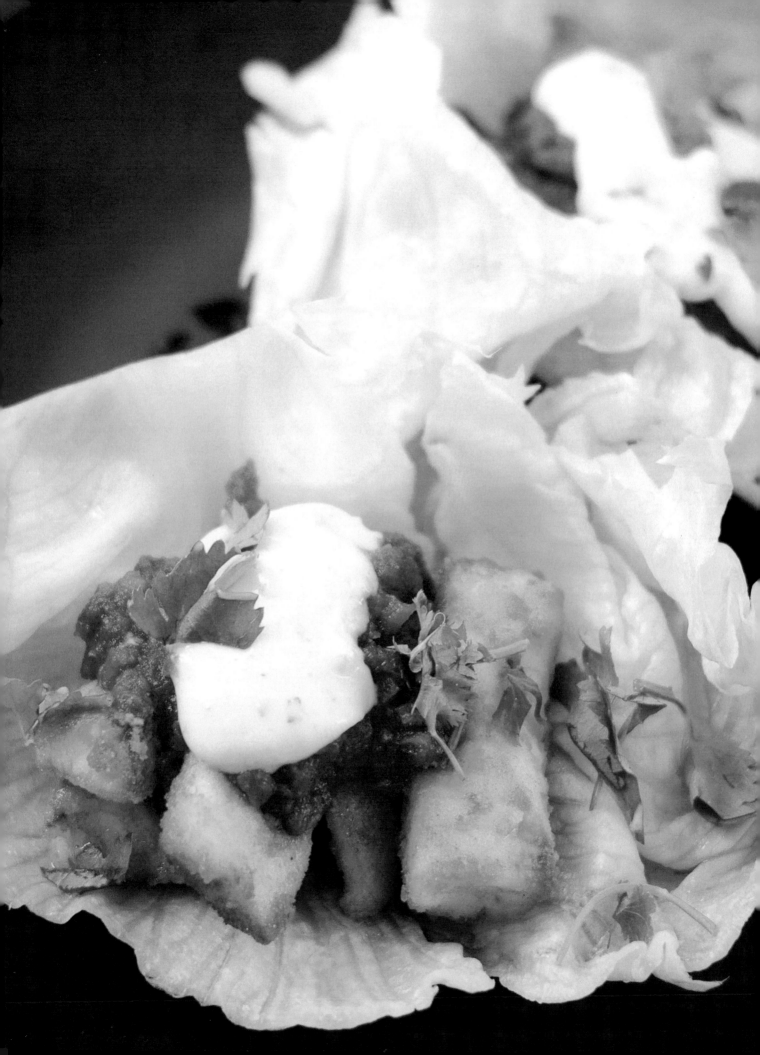

Fish Tacos with Plum Salsa

Prep Time: 30 minutes
Cook Time: 15 minutes
Total Time: 45 minutes
Yield: 2 servings
Serving Size: 2-3 tacos

INGREDIENTS

For the Fish:
- 1 lb *(454 g)* white fish, cut into 1/2 by 3/4 inch *(1 by 2 cm)* strips
- 1/2 cup *(56 g)* coconut flour
- 1 Tablespoon *(10 g)* garlic powder
- 2 teaspoons *(10 g)* salt
- Coconut oil *(for frying)*

For the White Sauce:
- 1/2 cup *(120 g)* coconut cream

For the Plum Salsa:
- 2 plums, diced small
- 1 teaspoon *(5 ml)* balsamic vinegar
- 1 teaspoon *(0.5 g)* cilantro, finely diced

To Eat:
- 4-6 lettuce leaves
- 2 Tablespoons *(2 g)* cilantro, chopped
- 4-6 slices of lime

INSTRUCTIONS

For the Plum Salsa:

1. Mix all plum salsa ingredients together with a fork.

For the Fish:

2. Mix together all dry ingredients *(coconut flour, garlic powder, salt)* in a bowl.

3. Drop the fish strips into the bowl and coat with the coconut flour mixture.

4. Heat up enough coconut oil in a saucepan so that the coconut oil is approx. 1/2 inch *(1-2 cm)* deep. Use a high heat.

5. Carefully add the coated fish strips to the hot coconut oil.

6. Fry until the coconut flour coating turns a golden brown color *(takes approx. 5 minutes)*. You should turn the fish strips over after a few minutes since the oil doesn't cover the entire piece of fish.

7. Place the fried fish strips in a bowl lined with a paper towel to soak up the excess oil.

To Eat:

8. Wash the lettuce leaves and pat dry with a paper towel.

9. Place 5-6 fish strips onto a lettuce leaf. Top with salsa and white sauce. Sprinkle some chopped cilantro on top for garnish and serve with a few slices of lime.

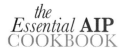

the **Essential AIP** COOKBOOK

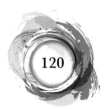

Mango Sashimi Salad

Prep Time: 15 minutes
Cook Time: 0 minutes
Total Time: 15 minutes
Yield: 2 servings
Serving Size: 1 plate

Try this salad with a side of Cold Cucumber Mash *(see Page 134 for recipe)* for something different.

INGREDIENTS
- 2 handfuls of baby kale leaves
- 1 Ataulfo mango, peeled and sliced
- 1/2 lb *(225 g)* salmon sashimi, sliced into 10-12 slices
- 1/2 Tablespoon *(7 g)* raw honey
- 3 Tablespoons *(45 ml)* coconut aminos
- 2 Tablespoons *(30 ml)* olive oil
- 1 teaspoon *(5 ml)* balsamic vinegar

INSTRUCTIONS
1. In a small bowl, mix together the honey, coconut aminos, olive oil, and balsamic vinegar to make the salad dressing.
2. Toss the dressing with the kale leaves in a large bowl, and then divide into 2 bowls.
3. Top each bowl of salad with mango slices and sashimi.

SUBSTITUTIONS
• Other salad leaves can be used instead of baby kale leaves.
• Smoked salmon can be used instead of salmon sashimi.
• Other types of mangoes or fruits can be used.

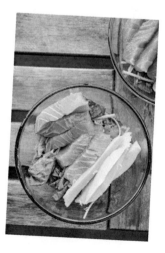

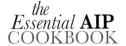

Rosemary Baked Salmon

Prep Time: 5 minutes
Cook Time: 30 minutes
Total Time: 35 minutes
Yield: 2 servings
Serving Size: 1 filet

Another recipe that we eat all the time. You can even use frozen salmon for this one *(although fresh is always a little tastier)*.

INGREDIENTS

- 2 salmon filets *(fresh or defrosted)*
- 1 Tablespoon *(2 g)* fresh rosemary leaves
- 1/4 cup *(60 ml)* olive oil
- 1 teaspoon *(6 g)* salt *(optional or to taste)*

INSTRUCTIONS

1. Preheat the oven to 350 F *(175 C)*.

2. Mix the olive oil, rosemary, and salt together in a bowl.

3. Place one salmon filet at a time into the mixture and rub the mixture onto the filet.

4. Wrap each filet in a piece of aluminum foil or parchment paper with some of the remaining mixture.

5. Bake for 25-30 minutes.

SUBSTITUTIONS

- Fresh or dried dill can be used instead of rosemary *(dried rosemary can also be used)*.

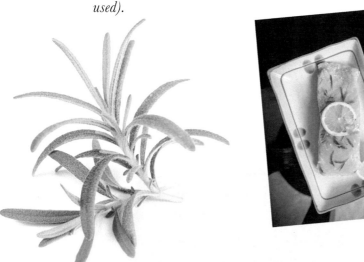

Chapter 3E:

Other

Blueberry Liver Stir-Fry

Prep Time: 10 minutes
Cook Time: 10 minutes
Total Time: 20 minutes
Yield: 1 serving
Serving Size: 1 plate

I know many people find the taste of liver to be a bit off-putting. But liver is highly nutritious so it's good to eat it regularly in your diet. And the blueberries in this recipe help to cover up some of the liver taste.

Enjoy with some Apple Bacon Brussels Sprouts *(see Page 131 for recipe)* as a side dish.

INGREDIENTS
- 1/2 lb *(225 g)* liver *(beef, chicken, or pork)*, diced
- 1 Tablespoon *(4 g)* scallions *(green onions)*, chopped finely
- 1/2 cup *(95 g)* blueberries
- 1 cup Swiss chard, chopped into small pieces
- 1 Tablespoon *(15 ml)* coconut oil *(to cook with)*
- Salt *(to taste)*

INSTRUCTIONS
1. Add the coconut oil to a pan on medium heat.
2. When the coconut oil is melted, add in the scallions followed by the liver.
3. Cook for a few minutes so that the liver starts to brown.
4. Add in the blueberries, followed by the Swiss chard.
5. Saute until the liver is cooked.
6. Add salt to taste.

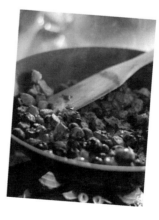

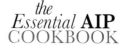

Italian Seasoning Crusted Lamb

Prep Time: 5 minutes
Cook Time: 30 minutes
Total Time: 35 minutes
Yield: 1 serving
Serving Size: 1 lamb steak

This is such an easy way to make flavorful and tender lamb steaks or lamb chops. The instructions are for baking in the oven, but you can also cook these on the grill. It's easy to double, triple, etc. this recipe - just adjust the cooking time depending on the thickness of the lamb.

You can make your own Italian seasoning for this recipe or check carefully that the ingredients are AIP-compliant.

Enjoy with some Rosemary Roasted Vegetables *(see Page 147 for recipe)*.

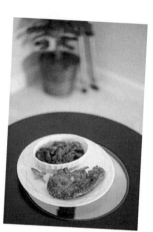

INGREDIENTS
- 1 lamb steak or chop *(0.5 lb or 250 g) (approx. 3/4-inch thick)*
- 1 Tablespoon *(3 g)* Italian Seasoning
- 2 Tablespoons *(20 g)* garlic powder
- Salt *(to taste)*

INSTRUCTIONS
1. Preheat oven to 375 F *(190 C)*.
2. Combine the Italian seasoning, garlic powder, and salt. Taste the mixture and adjust to taste.
3. Dip each lamb steak *(or lamb chop)* into the mixture and coat well.
4. Place on a baking tray and cook in the oven for 15 minutes. Then flip the lamb steak/chop and cook for another 15 minutes. This gets the lamb to around medium to medium well. Decrease or increase the cooking time for thinner or thicker steaks/chops or if you like your lamb rare or well done.

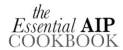

the
Essential **AIP**
COOKBOOK

Pressure Cooker Beet Cabbage Apple Stew

Prep Time: 10 minutes
Cook Time: 30 minutes
Total Time: 40 minutes
Yield: 4 servings
Serving Size: 1 bowl

I love how easy this veggie dish is - you can serve it either as a side dish or as an entree. If you don't have a pressure cooker, then make this in a large pot on the stove. You'll need to cook it for close to 1 hour until the beets have softened.

Enjoy some Oregano Raspberry Liver Pate *(see Page 142 for recipe)* and Garlic Crackers *(see Page 178 for recipe)* after your meal.

INGREDIENTS

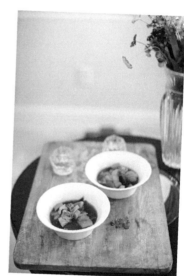

- 4 cups *(1 l)* chicken broth *(or bone broth)*
- 1 apple, diced
- 1/2 head of cabbage, chopped
- 1 small onion, chopped
- 2 beets *(164 g)*, chopped
- 2 small carrots *(100 g)*, chopped
- 1 Tablespoon fresh ginger *(5 g)*, grated
- 1 teaspoon *(2 g)* gelatin *(optional)*
- 2 Tablespoons *(4 g)* parsley
- Salt *(to taste)*

INSTRUCTIONS

1. Place everything into the pressure cooker. Cook on high pressure for 20 minutes. When ready, follow your pressure cooker's instructions for releasing the pressure safely.

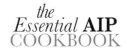

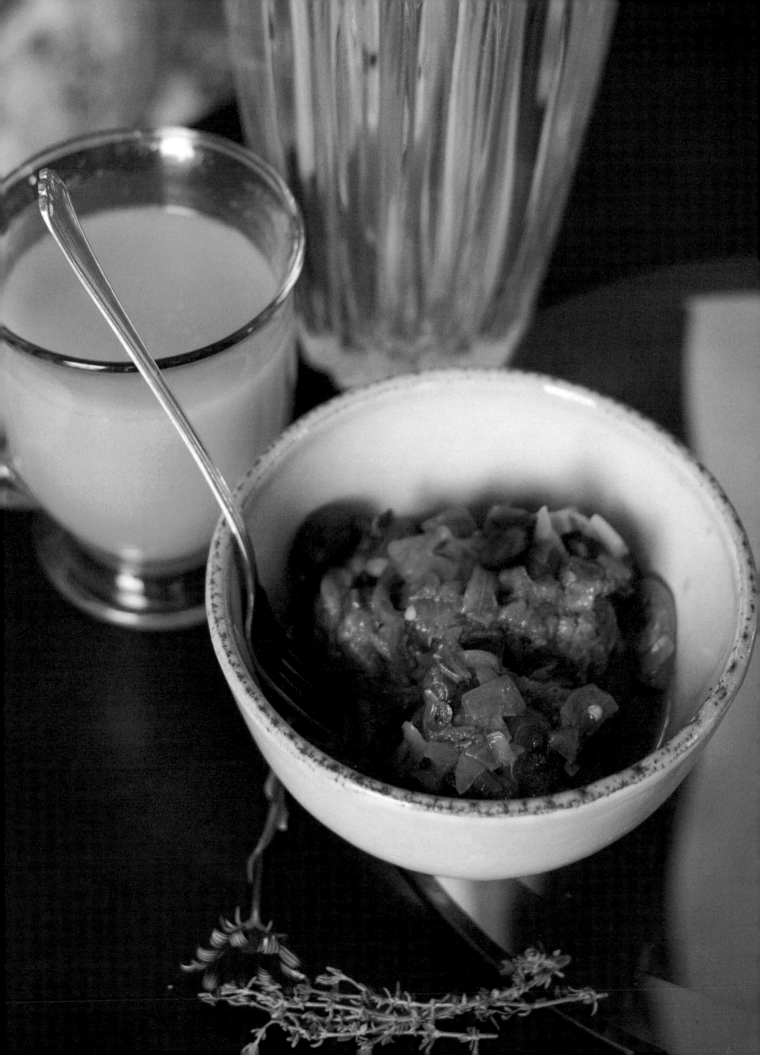

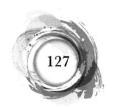

Pressure Cooker Jamaican Oxtail Stew

Prep Time: 15 minutes
Cook Time: 50 minutes
Total Time: 1 hour 5 minutes
Yield: 4 servings
Serving Size: 1 large bowl

If you don't have a pressure cooker, you can make this dish in the slow cooker - put it on the low setting for 8-10 hours and add more water so that it covers the meat. The meat should almost be falling off the bone when done.

Enjoy with some Cauliflower White "Rice" *(see Page 133 for recipe)* or some Fried Sweet Plantains *(see Page 139 for recipe)*.

INGREDIENTS
- 2 lbs *(900 g)* oxtail
- 1/2 large onion, chopped
- 2 green onions, chopped
- 6 cloves garlic, peeled
- 2 Tablespoons *(10 g)* fresh ginger, minced
- 1/4 cup *(60 ml)* coconut aminos
- 1 sprig thyme
- Salt *(to taste)*
- 2 cups *(480 ml)* water
- 2 Tablespoons *(30 ml)* avocado oil *(to cook with)*

INSTRUCTIONS
1. Place the avocado oil into a frying pan and add the chopped onions and oxtail. Cook the onions and oxtail on high heat until the outside of the oxtail starts to brown *(approx. 5-10 minutes)*. Stir regularly.
2. Place the browned oxtail and onions along with all the other ingredients into the pressure cooker.
3. Cook on high pressure for 50 minutes. When ready, follow your pressure cooker's instructions for releasing the pressure safely.

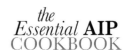

the
Essential **AIP**
COOKBOOK

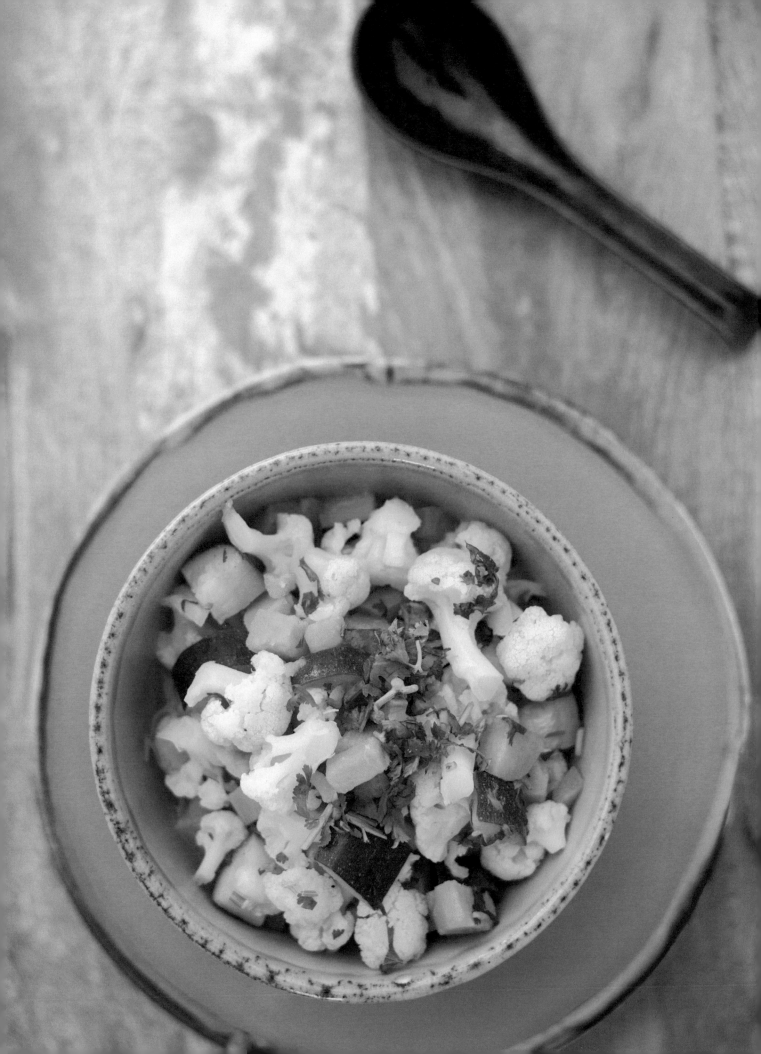

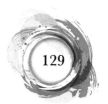

Turmeric Veggie "Curry"

Prep Time: 10 minutes
Cook Time: 20 minutes
Total Time: 30 minutes
Yield: 2 servings
Serving Size: 1 large bowl

Enjoy this "curry" by itself or with some Cauliflower White "Rice" *(see Page 133 for recipe)*, some Baked Spaghetti Squash *(see Page 132 for recipe)*, or some Garlic Cauliflower Naan Bread *(see Page 176 for recipe)*.

INGREDIENTS

- 2 cups *(480 ml)* broth *(or water)*
- 2 small sweet potatoes *(approx. 8 oz)*, peeled and diced
- 1/2 small cauliflower *(approx. 8 oz)*, broken into very small florets
- 1 zucchini, diced
- 1 Tablespoon *(3 g)* turmeric
- 1/2 Tablespoon *(5 g)* garlic powder
- 1/2 Tablespoon *(3.5 g)* onion powder
- 1/4 cup *(15 g)* cilantro, finely chopped
- Salt *(to taste)*
- 1 Tablespoon *(9 g)* arrowroot powder *(optional)* *(for thickening curry)*

INSTRUCTIONS

1. Place the broth in a saucepan and start boiling with the lid on. Add the turmeric, garlic powder, onion powder, and salt to taste and replace the lid.
2. Meanwhile, peel and then dice the sweet potatoes into very small chunks *(1/5-inch cubes)*. Place sweet potato cubes into saucepan and replace the lid.
3. Break the cauliflower into small florets and place into saucepan and replace the lid.
4. Dice the zucchini and place into saucepan and replace the lid.
5. Boil for 10 more minutes.
6. Add in the cilantro, mix well, and serve.
7. [OPTIONAL - to thicken the soup, remove the vegetables and keep the soup simmering on the stove. In a small bowl, mix 1 Tablespoon *(9 g)* of arrowroot powder with 2 Tablespoons *(30 ml)* cold water. Pour the mixture into the soup and stir for 1 minute until it thickens. Pour the thick soup over the vegetables.]

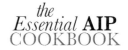

Chapter 4:
Side Dishes

Apple Bacon Brussels Sprouts

Prep Time: 10 minutes
Cook Time: 20 minutes
Total Time: 30 minutes
Yield: 2 servings
Serving Size: 1 large bowl

Bacon makes everything better, but when it comes to Brussels sprouts *(one of our favorite veggies)*, bacon is an almost magical addition. And it's even better when you cook the Brussels sprouts in the bacon fat. Try it and love it.

INGREDIENTS

- 1 lb *(454 g)* Brussels sprouts, finely chopped
- 1 medium apple, peeled and diced
- 2-3 slices of bacon, uncooked, chopped into small pieces
- Salt *(to taste)*

INSTRUCTIONS

1. Toss the bacon pieces into a large frying pan and let it cook until almost crispy.
2. Add in the Brussels sprouts and saute.
3. After 5 minutes, add in the apple pieces, and saute until the Brussels sprouts are as soft as you want it.
4. Add salt to taste.

SUBSTITUTIONS

• Another meat can be used instead of bacon like leftover short ribs from the Pressure Cooker Beef Short Ribs *(see Page 92 for recipe)*. Use coconut oil to cook the Brussels sprouts before adding in the leftover meat.
• A pear can be used instead of an apple.

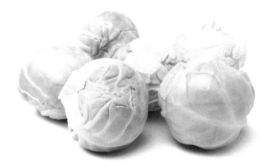

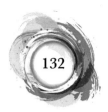

Baked Spaghetti Squash

Prep Time: 5 minutes
Cook Time: 45 minutes
Total Time: 50 minutes
Yield: 2 servings
Serving Size: 1 large plate

Baking spaghetti squash is easy, but if you don't have an oven, you can also make it in the microwave. Just remove the seeds, cover with coconut oil, and place in a shallow tray of water into the microwave *(7 minutes on high for each half)*. Make sure the water doesn't run out. You can also use this recipe to bake other squash.

If you have access to spaghetti squash, then give it a try as it's a fantastic AIP-friendly alternative to spaghetti.

INGREDIENTS
- 1 spaghetti squash
- 1 Tablespoon *(15 ml)* coconut oil

INSTRUCTIONS
1. Preheat oven to 375 F *(190 C)*.
2. Chop the spaghetti squash in half, remove seeds, cover inside of the spaghetti squash with coconut oil, place face down in a baking tray, and put into oven.
3. Bake for 45 minutes.
4. Use a fork to pull the spaghetti squash strands out of the squash.
5. Enjoy by itself or with some Beets "No-Tomato" Chili *(see Page 79 for recipe)* or some Turmeric Veggie "Curry" *(see Page 128 for recipe)*.

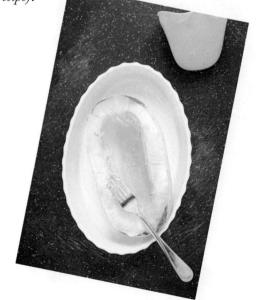

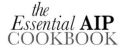

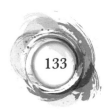

Cauliflower White "Rice"

Prep Time: 10 minutes
Cook Time: 15 minutes
Total Time: 25 minutes
Yield: 2 servings
Serving Size: 1 cup

This is the most basic of the cauliflower rice recipes - you can add your favorite meats and veggies to this recipe and create endless variations of your own. Or serve plain to go with a variety of entree dishes.

INGREDIENTS
- 1/2 head *(approx. 220 g)* cauliflower
- 1 Tablespoon *(15 ml)* coconut oil
- Salt *(to taste)*

INSTRUCTIONS
1. Cut up the cauliflower into small florets so that they'll fit into a food processor.
2. Process the cauliflower in the food processor until it forms very small "rice"-like pieces. Squeeze out excess water.
3. Add 1 Tablespoon *(15 ml)* of coconut oil into a large pot. Add in the cauliflower and let it cook on a medium heat. Stir regularly to make sure it doesn't burn!
4. Cook until tender but not mushy. Add salt to taste and serve.

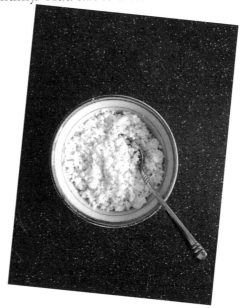

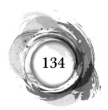

Cold Cucumber Mash

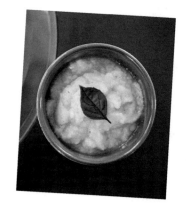

Prep Time: 15 minutes
Cook Time: 0 minutes
Total Time: 15 minutes
Yield: 1 serving
Serving Size: 1 cup

One of our favorite recipes during the summer is the simple cucumber salad *(chilled cucumber chunks with freshly minced garlic, olive oil, and salt)*. But for some more variation during the summer months, we started making this easy cucumber mash instead. It's refreshing and won't weigh you down at all!

INGREDIENTS

- 1 cucumber *(12 oz or 340 g)*, peeled and cut into large chunks
- 5 small *(or 3 large leaves)* basil leaves
- Juice from 1/4 lime
- 1/4 cup *(60 ml)* water *(to get blender going)*
- 1 teaspoon *(5 ml)* olive oil
- 1 teaspoon *(3 g)* garlic powder *(or to taste)*
- Salt *(to taste)*

INSTRUCTIONS

1. Place the cucumber, basil, lime juice, and water into a blender and blend well.
2. Using a strainer, squeeze the liquid out of the cucumber mash.
3. Mix in the olive oil, garlic powder, and salt.
4. Enjoy chilled!

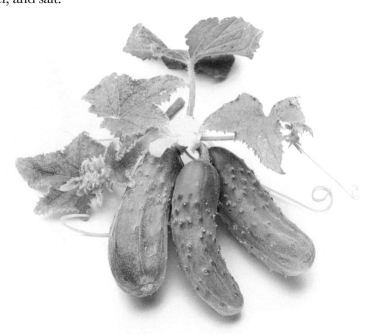

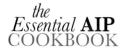

135

Creamy Cauliflower Mash

Prep Time: 20 minutes
Cook Time: 0 minutes
Total Time: 20 minutes
Yield: 2 servings
Serving Size: 1 small bowl

In fact, most people I've served this dish to were shocked to find that it's made using cauliflower as the texture and taste is just so smooth and creamy.

INGREDIENTS

- 1/2 head cauliflower *(approx 1.5 lb or 700 g)*, broken into small florets
- 2 Tablespoons *(30 ml)* coconut oil
- 1/4 cup *(60 ml)* coconut milk *(from a can shaken and at room temperature)*
- Chives or scallions *(spring onion)*, finely chopped *(optional)*
- Salt *(to taste)*

INSTRUCTIONS

1. Place the cauliflower florets into a large microwaveable bowl with 1/4 cup of water at the bottom. Microwave on high until they are softened *(around 10-12 minutes)*. Check every 3 minutes to make sure there's water in the bowl still. Alternatively, you can steam the cauliflower florets.
2. Place the softened cauliflower along with the coconut oil, coconut milk, and salt into a blender and blend until smooth.
3. Top with chives or scallions.

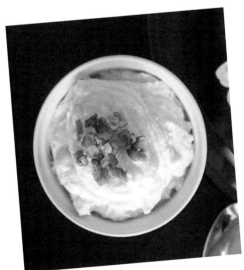

the Essential **AIP** COOKBOOK

Creamy Mashed Sweet Potatoes

Prep Time: 15 minutes
Cook Time: 30 minutes
Total Time: 45 minutes
Yield: 4 servings
Serving Size: 1 cup

Sometimes, it's the simplest dishes that you make over and over again, but also which really impress guests. This is one of those recipes - it's always the dish that empties most quickly.

INGREDIENTS

- 4 sweet potatoes
- 1 cup *(240 ml)* coconut cream *(or coconut milk)*
- 1 teaspoon *(2 g)* freshly grated ginger
- 2 Tablespoons *(10 g)* shredded coconut *(for topping)*

INSTRUCTIONS

1. Bake the sweet potatoes at 350 F *(175 C)* for about an hour. Or alternatively, boil the sweet potatoes for about 30 minutes. In either case, make sure the sweet potatoes are very tender - you should be able to poke a fork into them with ease. *(You can also microwave or steam the sweet potatoes to soften them.)*
2. Let the sweet potatoes cool for a bit and then peel them.
3. Place the peeled sweet potatoes into a food processor with the coconut cream and ginger, and food process on high until smooth.
4. Place the mashed sweet potatoes into a large bowl and top with shredded coconut.

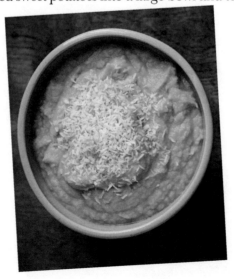

Easy Bacon Brussels Sprouts

Prep Time: 5 minutes
Cook Time: 20 minutes
Total Time: 25 minutes
Yield: 4-6 servings
Serving Size: 1 cup *(approx.)*

This is another recipe I make when guests come over - it's just so simple and yet so delicious!

INGREDIENTS

- 2 lbs *(908 g)* Brussels sprouts
- 1 lb *(454 g)* bacon, uncooked

INSTRUCTIONS

1. Boil the Brussels sprouts for 10 minutes until tender.
2. While the Brussels sprouts are boiling, chop the bacon into small pieces *(approx. 1/2-inch wide)*, and cook the bacon pieces in a large pot on medium heat. When the bacon is crispy, add in the drained Brussels sprouts.
3. Cook for 10 more minutes on high heat, mixing occasionally to make sure nothing gets burnt on the bottom of the pan.

SUBSTITUTIONS

• Another meat can be used instead of bacon like leftover short ribs from the Pressure Cooker Beef Short Ribs *(see Page 92 for recipe)*. Use coconut oil to cook the Brussels sprouts before adding in the leftover meat.

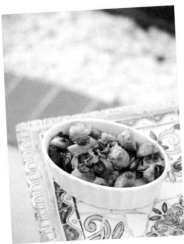
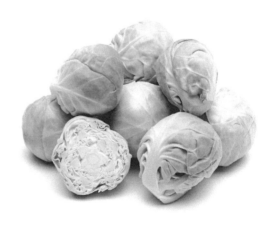

Endives and Pear Saute

Prep Time: 5 minutes
Cook Time: 10 minutes
Total Time: 15 minutes
Yield: 2 servings
Serving Size: 1 cup *(approx.)*

INGREDIENTS
- 4 Belgian endives, chopped into 1-inch chunks
- 1 pear, chopped into large chunks
- 2 cloves garlic, minced
- 1 teaspoon *(5 ml)* apple cider vinegar
- Salt *(to taste)*
- 1 Tablespoon *(15 ml)* coconut oil to cook with

INSTRUCTIONS
1. Place 1 Tablespoon of coconut oil into a frying pan on medium heat and add the endives.
2. When the endives start wilting a bit, add the minced garlic, pear pieces, vinegar, and salt to taste. Combine well.
3. Cook for 2 minutes and serve.

SUBSTITUTIONS
- Cabbage, Napa cabbage, or radicchio can be used instead of Belgian endives.

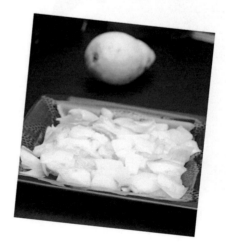

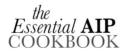

Fried Sweet Plantains

Prep Time: 10 minutes
Cook Time: 30 minutes
Total Time: 40 minutes
Yield: 2 servings
Serving Size: approx. 15 pieces

INGREDIENTS

- 2 ripe plantains
- 4 Tablespoons *(60 ml)* coconut oil *(for frying)*

INSTRUCTIONS

1. Peel the plantains and cut into 3 chunks lengthwise. Thinly slice each chunk to form long 4-5 thin strips *(not round slices)*.
2. Place 4 Tablespoons *(60 ml)* of coconut oil into pan on low heat.
3. Place the plantains strips into the pan and cook gently.
4. Flip the plantain strips after 10-15 minutes and cook the other side.
5. Keep cooking and turning for 30-40 minutes until the plantains are soft.

SUBSTITUTIONS

- Bananas can be used instead of plantains.

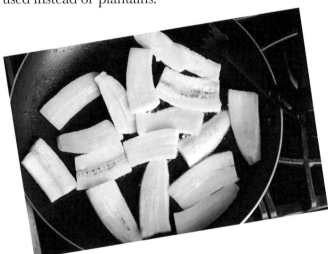

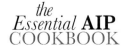

Garlic Lemon Broccolini Saute

Prep Time: 5 minutes
Cook Time: 10 minutes
Total Time: 15 minutes
Yield: 2 servings
Serving Size: 1 plate

I love a good green vegetable side dish especially with meats as the entree, and this one is simple and tasty. It's especially good as a side dish to steaks.

INGREDIENTS

- 1/2 lb *(225 g)* broccolini
- 3 cloves garlic, minced
- 1 Tablespoon *(15 ml)* lemon juice
- 1 Tablespoon *(10 g)* garlic powder *(optional)*
- 2 Tablespoons *(30 ml)* olive oil
- Salt *(to taste)*

INSTRUCTIONS

1. Add the olive oil into the saute pan on medium heat.
2. Add in the broccolini and saute for 5 minutes *(parboil the broccolini first if you prefer it softer)*.
3. Add in the minced garlic, lemon juice, garlic powder, and salt.
4. Saute for a few more minutes and serve immediately.

SUBSTITUTIONS

• Chopped broccoli can be used instead of broccolini.

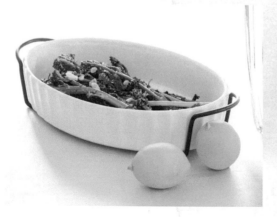

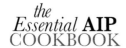

Ginger and Garlic Bok Choy Stir-Fry

Prep Time: 5 minutes
Cook Time: 10 minutes
Total Time: 15 minutes
Yield: 2 servings
Serving Size: 1 plate

INGREDIENTS

- 5 bok choy bunches
- 2 cloves of garlic, minced
- 1 teaspoon *(1.7 g)* fresh ginger, grated
- Salt *(to taste)*
- Coconut oil *(to cook in)*

INSTRUCTIONS

1. Cut off the ends of the bok choy. Then chop the bok choy into 1-inch long chunks.
2. Add 1 Tablespoon *(15 ml)* of coconut oil into a saucepan *(or wok)* on a medium heat, and then add in the bok choy chunks. Stir frequently while the bok choy cooks.
3. After the bok choy starts to wilt, mix in the garlic, ginger, and salt to taste.
4. Cook for another 1-2 minutes and serve.

SUBSTITUTIONS

- Other greens can be used instead of bok choy e.g., spinach.

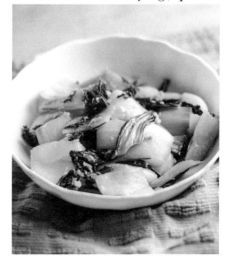

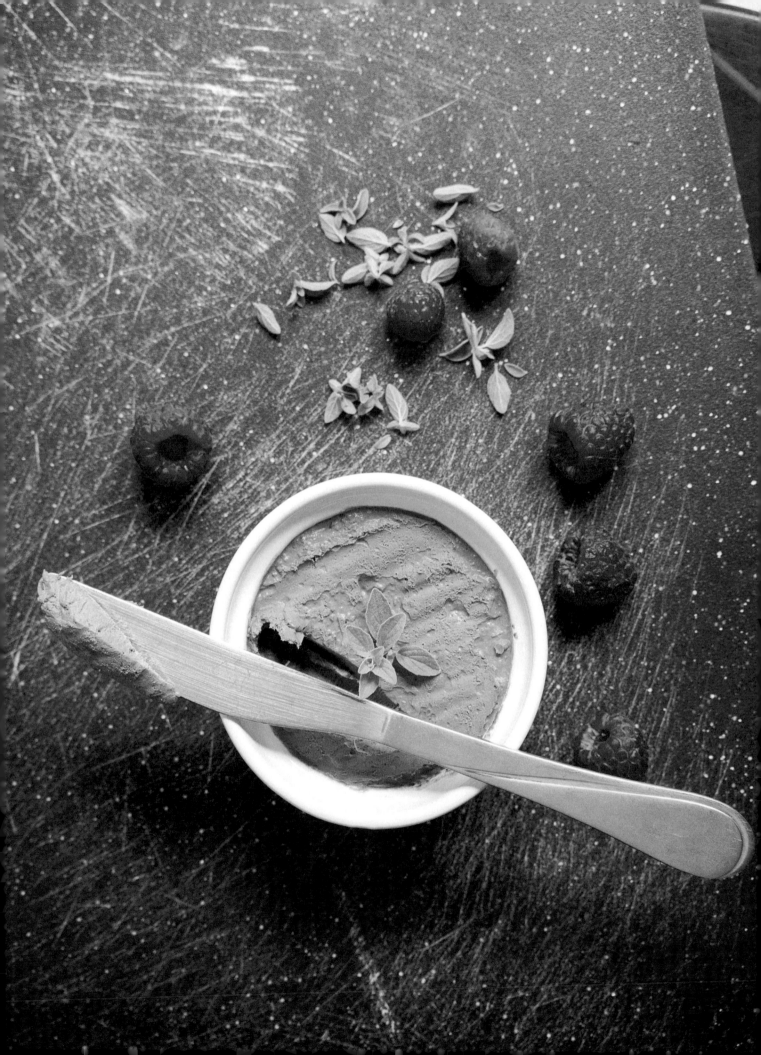

Oregano Raspberry Liver Pate

Prep Time: 10 minutes
Cook Time: 20 minutes
Total Time: 30 minutes
Yield: 4 servings
Serving Size: 2-3 Tablespoons

Liver is one of the healthiest foods you can eat, and chicken liver is easy to find. You can sneak liver into many of the meat dishes in the entree section or if you like the taste of liver, then make this simple liver pate.

I've included it as a Side Dish so you can serve it at any meal - try it with some Garlic Crackers *(see Page 178 for recipe)* or with the Garlic Cauliflower Naan Bread *(see Page 176 for recipe)*.

INGREDIENTS
- 0.7 lb *(320 g)* chicken liver
- 2 Tablespoons *(30 ml)* coconut oil *(may need extra)* *(or use olive oil)*
- 1/2 onion, chopped
- Approx. 50 oregano leaves
- 15 raspberries *(optional)* *(makes the pate less smooth)*
- Salt *(to taste)*

INSTRUCTIONS
1. Melt 2 Tablespoons of coconut oil in a pan and saute the chopped onions and chicken liver until the liver is cooked *(just pink inside)*. This takes 10-15 minutes on medium heat, and you may find putting a lid onto the pan for 5 minutes at the end helps.
2. Add in the oregano leaves a few minutes before the liver is done.
3. Blend the liver, onions, oregano, raspberries, and salt until smooth *(add in an extra Tablespoon of coconut oil if needed to make the pate smoother)*.

SUBSTITUTIONS
- Other herbs and berries can be used instead of the oregano and raspberries.

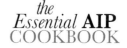

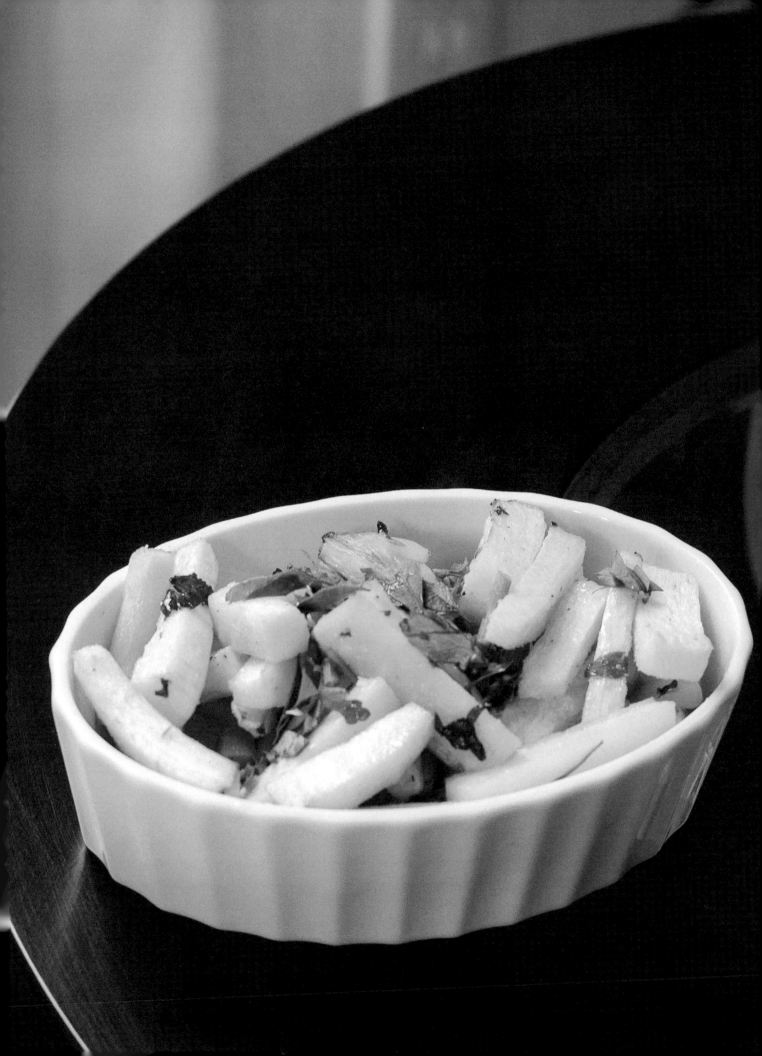

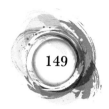

Super Fast Avocado Salad

Prep Time: 5 minutes
Cook Time: 0 minutes
Total Time: 5 minutes
Yield: 1 serving
Serving Size: 1 cup

INGREDIENTS

- 1 ripe avocado
- 1 Tablespoon *(15 ml)* olive oil
- 1 Tablespoon *(15 ml)* balsamic vinegar
- Salt *(to taste)*

INSTRUCTIONS

1. Cut a ripe avocado in half.
2. Remove the pit, and using a small knife carefully score each half into cubes. Then use a spoon to scoop out the avocado - it'll be in nice cubes now.
3. Toss the avocado cubes with olive oil, balsamic vinegar, and salt.

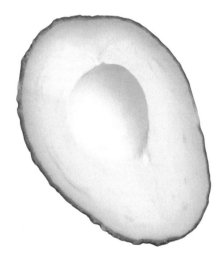

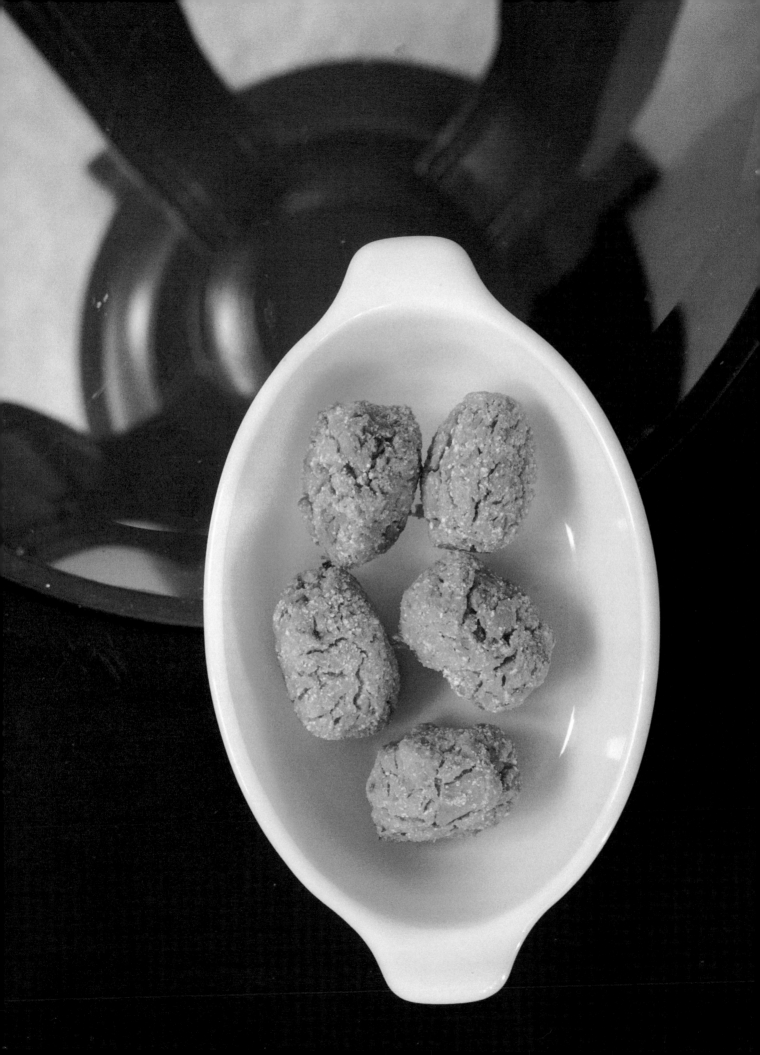

Sweet Potato Tater Tots

Prep Time: 15 minutes
Cook Time: 30 minutes
Total Time: 45 minutes
Yield: 4 servings
Serving Size: 10-15 tater tots

INGREDIENTS

- 2 large sweet potatoes *(approx. 4 cups (532 g))*, peeled and cubed
- 4 Tablespoons *(28 g)* coconut flour
- 1/2 teaspoon *(3 g)* salt

INSTRUCTIONS

1. Preheat the oven to 425 F *(220 C)*.

2. Steam the sweet potato cubes until just soft *(approx. 15 minutes – you don't want them too soft)*. Alternatively, bake or microwave the sweet potatoes.

3. In a food processor or blender, mix together the sweet potatoes *(make sure they're not too hot and pour out any water from the steamer)*, coconut flour, and salt.

4. Form the mixture into small balls *(with your hands or a mini ice-cream scoop or a spoon)*.

5. Place the balls onto a parchment paper lined baking sheet and bake for 15 minutes.

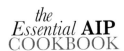

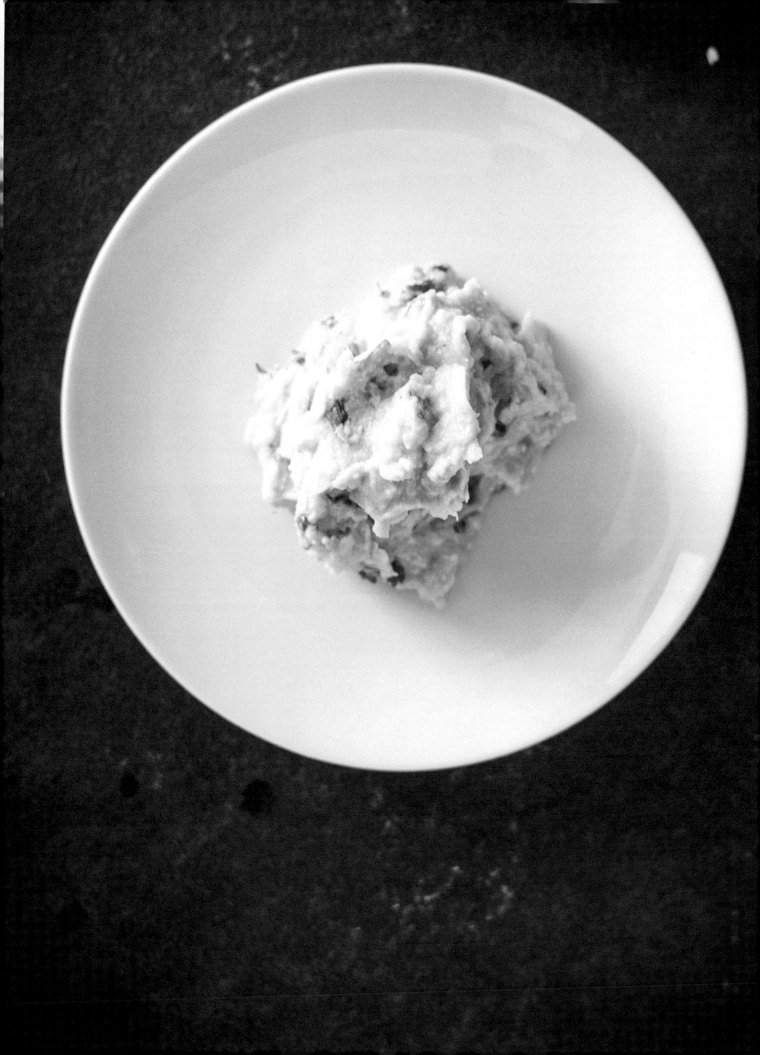

5-Min Super Easy Guacamole

Prep Time: 5 minutes
Cook Time: 0 minutes
Total Time: 5 minutes
Yield: 2 servings
Serving Size: 1 small bowl

This guacamole not only omits the tomatoes and peppers but is super quick and easy to make. Enjoy it with some grilled steak or chicken for a quick and easy meal.

INGREDIENTS

- 1 ripe avocado, mashed
- 1 Tablespoon *(10 g)* garlic powder
- 1/2 Tablespoon *(3.5 g)* onion powder
- 2 teaspoons *(10 ml)* lime juice
- Salt *(to taste)*
- 2 Tablespoons *(4 g)* fresh cilantro, finely chopped *(or use 2 teaspoons (2 g) of dried cilantro)*

INSTRUCTIONS

1. Mash up the avocado. Make sure your avocado is ripe as it won't make very good guacamole otherwise.
2. Mix in 1 Tablespoon of garlic powder and 1/2 Tablespoon of onion powder.
3. Squeeze in the fresh lime juice and finely chopped cilantro.
4. Mix everything together really well. Add salt to taste and serve.

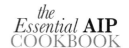

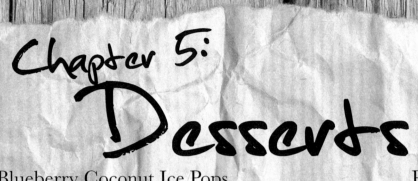

Chapter 5: Desserts

Blueberry Coconut Ice Pops

Prep Time: 10 minutes
Cook Time: 0 minutes
Total Time: 10 minutes + 4 hours freezing time
Yield: 2 servings
Serving Size: 1 *(2.5 oz)* ice pop

INGREDIENTS

- 1/2 cup *(95 g)* blueberries
- 1/4 cup *(60 ml)* coconut milk
- 1 teaspoon *(7 g)* raw honey
- 1 Tablespoon *(15 ml)* lemon juice
- Pinch of salt

INSTRUCTIONS

1. Blend all the ingredients together well.

2. Taste the mixture and add more of any ingredient you want.

3. Pour into ice pop molds *(this recipe makes two 2.5 oz bars)*. Make sure there's a bit of space left over as the mixture will expand when it freezes.

4. Freeze for 4+ hours. When ready to eat, run the ice pop mold for a few minutes under hot water to make it easier to pull the ice pops out.

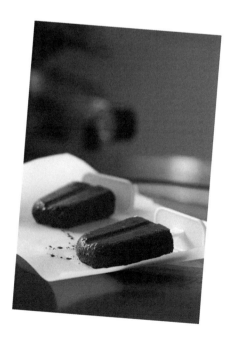

Boiled Bananas in Coconut Milk

Prep Time: 2 minutes
Cook Time: 10 minutes
Total Time: 12 minutes
Yield: 2 servings
Serving Size: 1 bowl

I first saw this recipe in Vietnam, and I was struck by how AIP-friendly it was! There are of course many variations of it throughout Asia, but I've created a simple version below with AIP-friendly ingredients.

INGREDIENTS
- 2 bananas, peeled
- 2 cups *(480 ml)* coconut milk
- Raw honey *(to taste)*

INSTRUCTIONS
1. Cut the bananas into 1-inch thick chunks.
2. Place the coconut milk into a small saucepan and boil it.
3. Once the coconut milk is boiling, add the banana chunks to the coconut milk and simmer for 5 minutes.
4. Place into a bowl and drizzle with raw honey if desired.

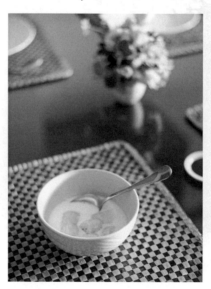

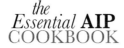
the Essential **AIP** COOKBOOK

Coconut Pan-Fried Pineapple

Prep Time: 5 minutes
Cook Time: 5 minutes
Total Time: 10 minutes
Yield: 2-4 servings
Serving Size: 1-2 pineapple slices

Fruit makes wonderfully easy desserts. And the best thing is you don't have to do much to them. If you've never tried adding salt on pineapple, give it a try *(just add a pinch)*. It's really good! Cinnamon also works really well with pineapple.

INGREDIENTS

- 2-4 pineapple slices
- 2 Tablespoons *(30 ml)* coconut oil
- Sea salt *(to taste) (optional)*
- 1/2 lime *(optional)*

INSTRUCTIONS

1. Cut off the pineapple skin and slice the pineapple into 1/2-inch to 1-inch thick round slices and remove the core.
2. Place the coconut oil into a frying pan on high heat *(or you can grill the pineapple)*.
3. Place the pineapple slices into the frying pan and fry for 2 minutes on each side.
4. Put each pineapple slice on a plate and squeeze a bit of lime juice and sprinkle some sea salt on top for extra flavor.

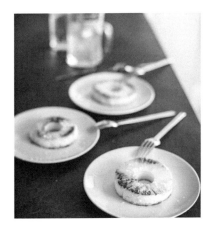

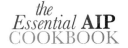

Carrot Gummies

Prep Time: 5 minutes
Cook Time: 5 minutes + 2 hours set time
Total Time: 2 hours 10 minutes
Yield: 6-8 servings
Serving Size: 2 large gummies

INGREDIENTS

- 2 cups *(480 ml)* carrot juice with some of the pulp
- 5 Tablespoons *(35 g)* gelatin powder

INSTRUCTIONS

1. Place the carrot juice into a small pot on the stove.
2. Heat on medium heat until the liquid starts to simmer.
3. Stir in the gelatin powder *(adding a small amount at a time)* until it's all dissolved.
4. Use a strainer to strain the liquid to remove any lumps that might have formed.
5. Pour into silicone molds *(ice cube trays work well)* and refrigerate for 2 hours.

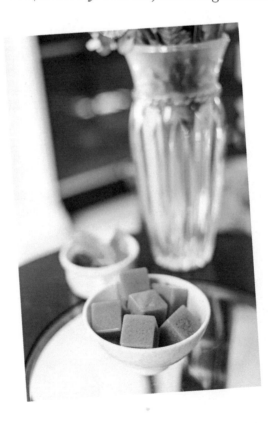

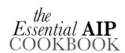

Coconut Banana Balls

Prep Time: 10 minutes
Cook Time: 15 minutes
Total Time: 25 minutes
Yield: 4 servings
Serving Size: 3 coconut balls

INGREDIENTS

- 1 banana, mashed
- 2 cups *(160 g)* unsweetened shredded coconut
- 1 Tablespoon *(21 g)* raw honey
- 2 Tablespoons *(30 ml)* coconut oil, melted
- Dash of salt
- Carob powder *(to sprinkle on top)*

INSTRUCTIONS

1. Preheat oven to 250 F *(120 C)* if serving warm.

2. Mix all the ingredients together in a bowl.

3. Form around 12 small balls *(1-inch diameter)* from the dough using your hands.

4. Refrigerate or bake at 250 F for 15 min.

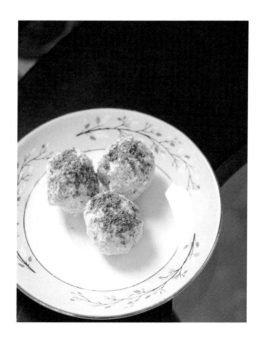

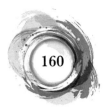

Coconut Butter Stuffed Dates

Prep Time: 10 minutes
Cook Time: 0 minutes
Total Time: 10 minutes
Yield: 2-3 servings
Serving: 5 dates

If you don't have coconut butter, you can make your own (read this article - http://paleomagazine.com/how-to-make-coconut-butter).

INGREDIENTS
- 10 pitted dates
- 1 cup *(250 g)* coconut butter

INSTRUCTIONS
1. Melt the coconut butter slightly in the microwave if it's not soft enough to scoop out with a spoon *(make sure to take the metal lid off the jar first before microwaving)*.
2. Slice open each date so that it opens out but isn't sliced in half.
3. Stuff each date with as much coconut butter as you can fit in while still being able to close it up.

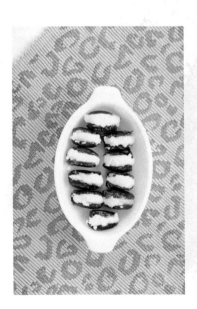

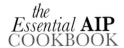

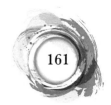

Easy Strawberry Ice Cream

Prep Time: 10 minutes
Cook Time: 0 minutes
Total Time: 10 minutes + 4 hours freezing time
Yield: 2 servings
Serving Size: 1/2-1 cup

INGREDIENTS

- 1 cup *(125 g)* fresh strawberries
- Coconut cream from the top of a refrigerated can *(14 oz)* of coconut milk *(approx. 1 cup or 240 ml)*
- 1 Tablespoon *(21 g)* raw honey
- Coconut flakes *(for sprinkling on top)*

INSTRUCTIONS

1. Blend the strawberries, coconut cream, and honey together in a blender *(you might need to melt the coconut cream and honey slightly depending on how cold your kitchen is)*.

2. Place the mixture into your ice cream maker and follow its instructions for making ice cream.

3. If you're not using an ice cream maker, then pour the mixture into a large bowl and place into the freezer. Stir the mixture every 30 minutes for 3-4 hours until it forms an ice cream consistency.

4. Sprinkle coconut flakes on top when serving.

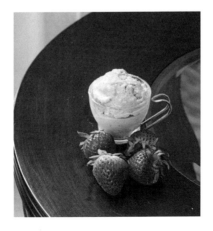

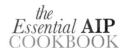

Honeyed Apples

Prep Time: 5 minutes
Cook Time: 10 minutes
Total Time: 15 minutes
Yield: 2 servings
Serving Size: 1/2 cup

INGREDIENTS

- 1 apple, peeled and diced
- 2 Tablespoons *(30 ml)* coconut oil
- 1/2 Tablespoon *(7 ml)* lime juice *(optional)*
- Drizzle of raw honey *(approx. 1 teaspoon or to taste)*

INSTRUCTIONS

1. Melt the coconut oil in a saucepan. Add in the diced apples, lime juice, and honey.
2. Cook for 10 minutes on medium heat until the apples soften.

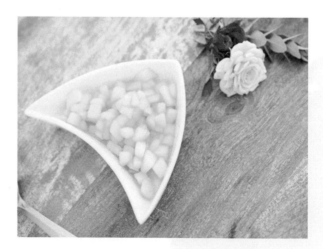

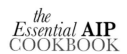

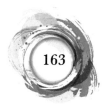
Mango Ginger Coconut Ice Cream

Prep Time: 15 minutes
Cook Time: 0 minutes
Total Time: 15 minutes
Yield: approx. 2 servings
Serving Size: 1 small ramekin

INGREDIENTS

- 1 cup *(220 g)* frozen mango chunks
- 1/4 cup *(60 ml)* coconut cream
- 1/4 cup *(20 g)* unsweetened shredded coconut
- 1/2 Tablespoon *(7 ml)* lime juice
- 1 teaspoon *(1.7 g)* ginger, grated *(as topping)*
- 2 Tablespoons *(42 g)* raw honey

INSTRUCTIONS

1. Let the mango chunks defrost for 5 minutes at room temperature.
2. Blend the mango, coconut cream, shredded coconut, lime juice, and raw honey well.
3. Top with the grated ginger.

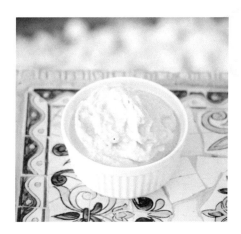

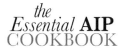

Mini Pumpkin Pie

Prep Time: 5 minutes
Cook Time: 0 minute
Total Time: 5 minutes
Yield: 1 serving
Serving Size: 1 ramekin

INGREDIENTS

- 6 Tablespoons *(100 g)* pumpkin puree
- 3 Tablespoons *(45 ml)* coconut oil
- 3 Tablespoons *(15 g)* carob powder
- Dash of cinnamon
- Dash of ginger powder
- Raw honey *(to taste)*

INSTRUCTIONS

1. Place all ingredients into a microwaveable bowl and microwave on high for approx. 45 seconds *(just to make it easier to blend)*.

2. Blend well.

3. Serve immediately warm, or chill in refrigerator for a more solid consistency.

4. Sprinkle a bit of carob powder on top before serving *(optional)*.

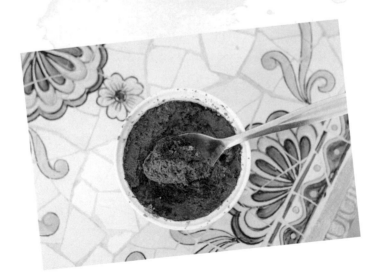

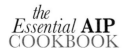

Pineapple Mango Banana Sorbet

Prep Time: 5 minutes
Cook Time: 0 minutes
Total Time: 5 minutes
Yield: 2 servings
Serving Size: 1 small bowl

INGREDIENTS

- 1/2 cup *(4 oz or 125 g)* frozen pineapples
- 1 cup *(8 oz or 250 g)* frozen mango pieces
- 1 banana *(room temperature)*
- 1 Tablespoon *(21 g)* raw honey *(optional)*
- 1/2 Tablespoon *(7 ml)* fresh lime juice
- 1 banana *(for topping) (optional)*

INSTRUCTIONS

1. Place all the ingredients *(except the banana for the topping)* into a blender and blend really well. Depending on how good your blender is, you may have to blend briefly and then push the frozen fruit down and repeat several times.
2. Top with a few banana slices.
3. Serve immediately.

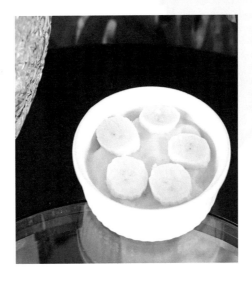

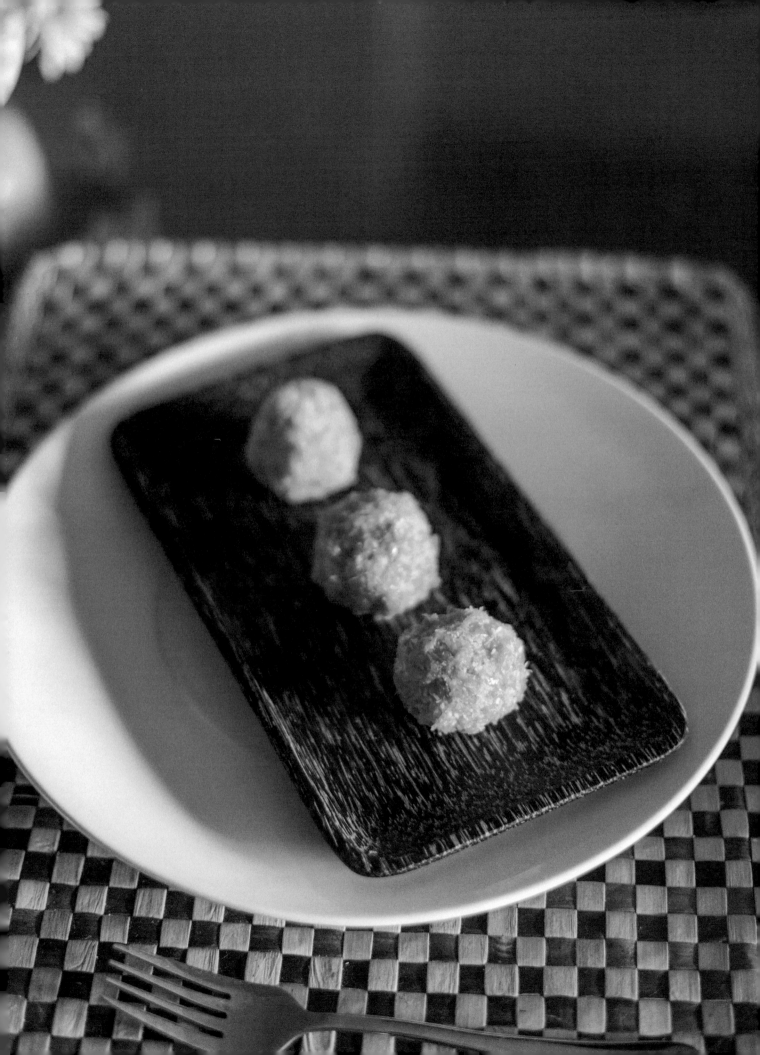

Raw Carrot Coconut Cake Bites

Prep Time: 5 minutes
Cook Time: 0 minutes
Total Time: 5 minutes + 1 hour in fridge
Yield: 2 servings
Serving Size: 2-3 bites

INGREDIENTS

- 1 cup *(100 g)* shredded carrot
- 1/2 cup *(40 g)* shredded coconut
- 1.5 Tablespoons *(28 g)* raw honey
- 1.5 Tablespoons *(22.5 ml)* coconut oil
- 1/2 teaspoon *(2 g)* cinnamon powder

INSTRUCTIONS

1. Squeeze out excess water from the carrots and then mix all ingredients together in a bowl.

2. Make into small balls *(4-6 balls)* and refrigerate for 1 hour before serving.

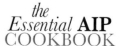

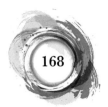

Sinh To Bo (Vietnamese Smoothie)

Prep Time: 5 minutes
Cook Time: 0 minutes
Total Time: 5 minutes
Yield: 1 serving
Serving Size: 1 glass

INGREDIENTS

- 1 avocado
- 1 cup *(240 g)* ice
- 1/2 cup *(120 ml)* coconut milk *(add a little bit more if you have trouble getting the mixture to blend)*
- 1 Tablespoon *(21 g)* raw honey *(add more to taste)*

INSTRUCTIONS

1. Cut a ripe avocado in half.
2. Use a spoon to scoop out the avocado flesh.
3. Place the avocado flesh into the blender with the ice, coconut milk, and honey, and blend well *(start slow and increase the speed slowly)*.
4. Add more coconut milk if necessary to blend until smooth.

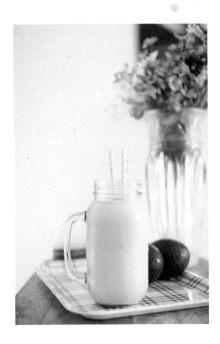

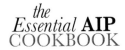

Strawberry & Blueberry Jello

Prep Time: 10 minutes
Cook Time: 0 minutes
Total Time: 10 minutes + 3 hours for setting
Yield: 2 servings
Serving: 1 cup

INGREDIENTS

- 1 cup *(125 g)* strawberries
- 1 cup *(130 g)* blueberries
- 2 Tablespoons *(14 g)* gelatin powder
- 1 cup *(240 ml)* of water

INSTRUCTIONS

1. Puree the strawberries and blueberries.

2. Pour the pureed fruit into cups, filling each cup half way.

3. Place 2 Tablespoons of the gelatin powder into a large bowl and add in 1 cup of cold water. Stir well. Then place the bowl into the microwave and heat on high for 1 minute. Mix well using a fork.

4. Pour the gelatin water into the cups with the fruit puree *(almost filling each cup to the brim)* and mix well.

5. Leave in the fridge to set for 3-4 hours.

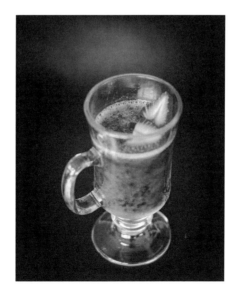

Thai Fried Bananas

Prep Time: 10 minutes
Cook Time: 10 minutes
Total Time: 20 minutes
Yield: 2 servings
Serving Size: 3 slices

I've found that many traditional Asian desserts happen to be very AIP-friendly naturally, so here is another great dessert.

For a full Thai dinner, serve these fried bananas after eating Thai Chicken Pad See Ew *(see Page 76 for recipe)*.

INGREDIENTS

- 1 ripe banana
- 3 Tablespoons *(45 ml)* coconut oil
- Raw honey *(optional)*

For the batter:
- 1/4 cup *(36 g)* tapioca flour or arrowroot powder
- 1 Tablespoon *(7 g)* coconut flour
- 1 teaspoon *(7 g)* raw honey *(optional)*
- 2-3 Tablespoons *(30-45 ml)* water

INSTRUCTIONS

1. Make the batter by mixing together all the batter ingredients to make a thick paste.
2. Slice the banana in half and then into thin slices lengthwise.
3. Place the coconut oil into a frying pan on hot heat.
4. Dip the banana slices into the batter, coat it and drop immediately into the coconut oil *(the batter comes off easily)*.
5. Fry until golden.
6. Place on paper towels to soak up the oil. Drizzle with honey *(optional)* and serve.

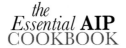

Ginger Baked Pear

Prep Time: 5 minutes
Cook Time: 1 hour
Total Time: 1 hour 5 minutes
Yield: 2 servings
Serving Size: 1 pear

INGREDIENTS

- 2 Bartlett/Williams pears
- 1.5 Tablespoon *(31.5 g)* honey
- 1.5 Tablespoon *(22.5 ml)* coconut oil
- 2 teaspoons *(2 g)* ginger powder
- 1 teaspoon *(5 ml)* lemon juice

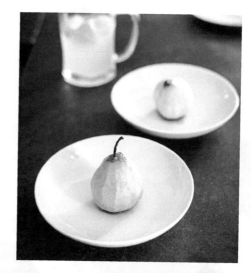

INSTRUCTIONS

1. Preheat oven to 400 F *(200 C)*.
2. Mix together the honey, coconut oil, ginger powder, and lemon juice in a small bowl.
3. Peel the pears and make sure they can stand by themselves on a baking tray. If not, then cut off a slice on the bottom of the pear to make it flat so that it can stand.
4. Use your hands *(or a spoon or a brush)* to cover the pears with the mixture. You should only need to use a very small amount of mixture to cover the pears *(around 1/4 of the mixture)*.
5. Place aluminum foil or parchment paper on a baking tray and place the pears on the tray and bake for 1 hour.
6. After 15 minutes, use a spoon to pour a bit more of the mixture on each pear. After 30 minutes in the oven, pour a bit more mixture on each pear. Continue baking for the last 30 minutes until the pear is pretty soft *(you should be able to cut it with a spoon)*.
7. Save the rest of the mixture to serve with.

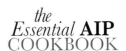

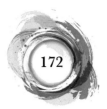

Tropical Fruit Salad

Prep Time: 10 minutes
Cook Time: 0 minutes
Total Time: 10 minutes
Yield: 2 servings
Serving Size: 1 cup

You can make this topical fruit salad 2 ways *(as an appetizer or as a dessert)* and you can use different fruits if you have trouble finding these delicious tropical ones.

INGREDIENTS

- Mango *(ripe, but not too soft) (4 oz or 125 g)*
- Papaya *(4 oz or 125 g)*
- Pineapple *(4 oz or 125 g)*
- 2 Tablespoons *(10 g)* coconut flakes
- 1/2 Tablespoon *(7 ml)* balsamic vinegar
- 2 Tablespoons *(30 ml)* olive oil

INSTRUCTIONS

1. Dice all the fruits into similar sized chunks.
2. Place the fruits together in a bowl and toss with balsamic vinegar and olive oil.
3. Sprinkle coconut flakes on top.

SUBSTITUTIONS

• For a sweeter option, switch the balsamic vinegar and olive oil for coconut cream instead.

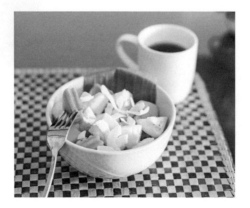

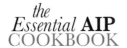

Chapter 6:

Snacks & Breads

Coconut Tea Gummies

Prep Time: 5 minutes
Cook Time: 5 minutes + 2 hours set time
Total Time: 2 hours 10 minutes
Yield: 6-8 servings
Serving Size: 2 large gummies

You can eat these gummies by themselves to get extra gelatin into your diet or chop these up into small pieces and add them to cold drinks like the Coconut Iced Tea Latte *(see Page 184 for recipe)* to make an Asian-style bubble or boba tea.

INGREDIENTS

- 2 cups *(480 ml)* black tea
- 3 Tablespoons *(45 ml)* coconut milk *(or to taste)*
- Raw honey *(to taste)*
- 5 Tablespoons *(35 g)* gelatin powder

INSTRUCTIONS

1. Place the tea, coconut milk, and honey into a small pot on the stove.
2. Heat on medium heat until the liquid starts to simmer.
3. Stir in the gelatin powder *(adding a small amount at a time)* until it's all dissolved.
4. Use a strainer to strain the liquid to remove any lumps that might have formed.
5. Pour into silicone molds *(ice cube trays work well)* and refrigerate for 2 hours to set.

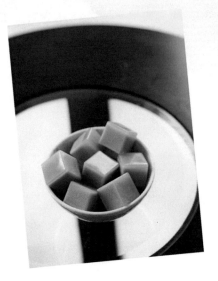

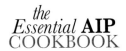

the
Essential **AIP**
COOKBOOK

Bread Rolls

Prep Time: 10 minutes
Cook Time: 50 minutes
Total Time: 1 hour
Yield: 2 servings
Serving Size: 1 bread roll

These bread rolls are denser than regular bread. Enjoy with some soups or stews.

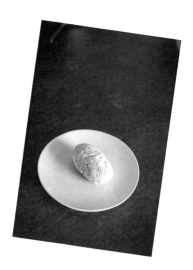

INGREDIENTS

- 2 Tablespoons *(30 ml)* coconut oil, melted
- 6 Tablespoons *(42 g)* coconut flour
- 1/4 teaspoon *(1 g)* baking soda
- 1 Tablespoon *(3 g)* Italian seasoning
- 1/2 teaspoon *(2.5 g)* salt
- 2 Tablespoons *(14 g)* gelatin
- 6 Tablespoons *(90 ml)* hot water

INSTRUCTIONS

1. Preheat the oven to 300 F *(150 C)*.
2. Mix together the coconut oil, coconut flour, and baking soda.
3. In a separate bowl, whisk together the gelatin and hot water to create your gelatin egg.
4. Pour the gelatin egg into the coconut flour mixture and combine well.
5. Add in the Italian seasoning and salt to taste *(you can taste the mixture to see if you want to add more)* and mix well into a dough.
6. Use your hands to form 2 small rolls from the dough, place the rolls on a baking tray lined with parchment paper, and bake in the oven for 40-50 minutes until the outside of each roll is slightly browned and crispy like you'd typically find in a regular bread roll.
7. Let the rolls cool down before serving so that the gelatin sets a bit and can hold the roll together. Enjoy at room temperature with some coconut oil.
8. This recipe can be doubled, tripled, etc. if you want to make more bread rolls at the same time.

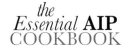

the
Essential **AIP**
COOKBOOK

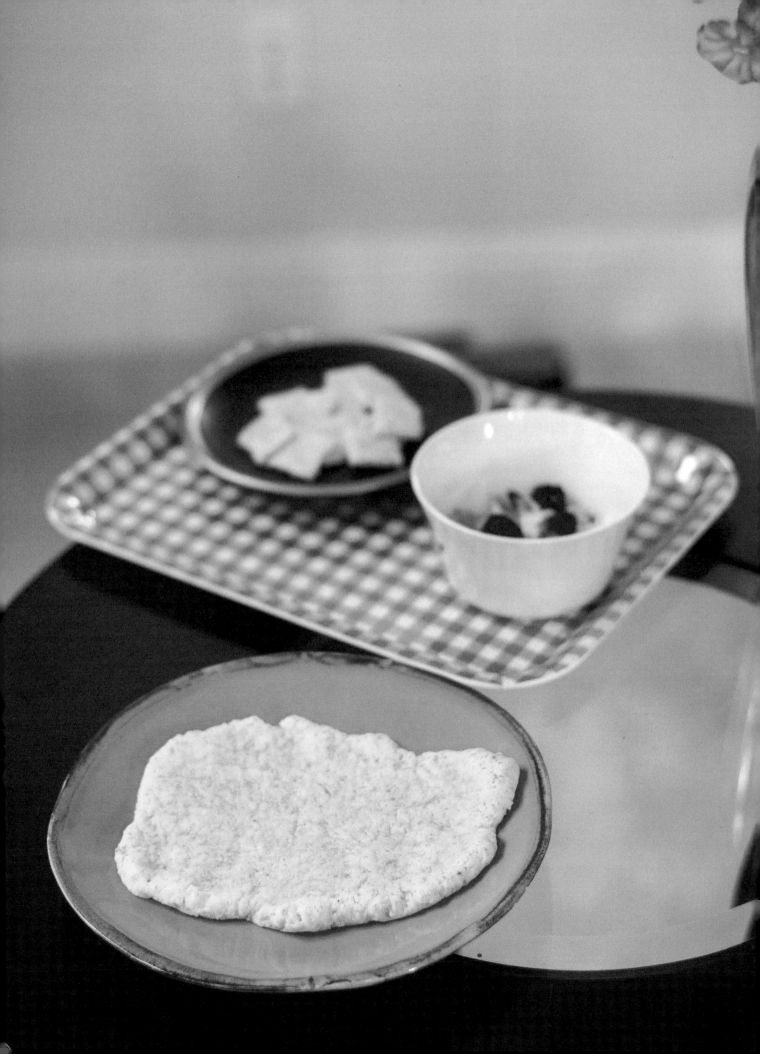

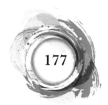

Garlic Cauliflower Naan Bread

Prep Time: 10 minutes
Cook Time: 15 minutes
Total Time: 25 minutes
Yield: 1 serving
Serving Size: 1 naan bread

This is one my favorite AIP recipes - this bread is stretchy and delicious in taste. Use it as a wrap (it doesn't fall apart easily) or dip it into stews.

INGREDIENTS

- 1 cup *(140 g)* cauliflower florets
- 1/2 cup *(64g)* arrowroot flour
- 1 Tablespoon *(7 g)* garlic powder
- 2 Tablespoons *(30 ml)* avocado oil
- Salt *(to taste)*

INSTRUCTIONS

1. Preheat oven to 450 F *(230 C)*.
2. Place the cauliflower florets into a bowl with some water and microwave on high until tender *(check every 2 minutes to make sure it doesn't burn)*. Alternatively, steam the florets until tender.
3. Food process *(or use a blender)* to process the cauliflower florets into a mash.
4. Mix the cauliflower mash with the arrowroot flour, garlic powder, avocado oil, and salt. Taste the mixture and add in more garlic powder and salt to taste. Mix into a springy dough.
5. Use your hands to press the dough into a flat bread, place on some parchment paper, and bake in oven for 15 minutes.
6. Let cool and serve.

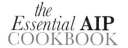

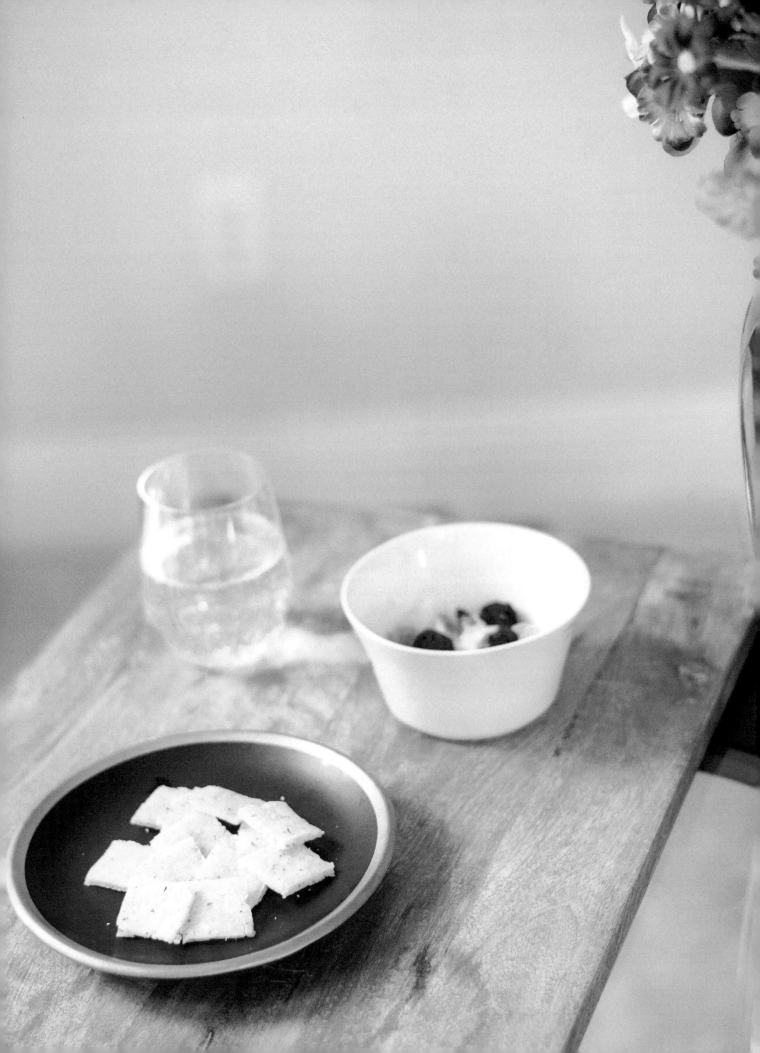

Garlic Crackers

Prep Time: 10 minutes
Cook Time: 15 minutes
Total Time: 25 minutes
Yield: 2 servings
Serving Size: 5-7 crackers *(approx.)*

These crackers are very crunchy! Give them a try with some Oregano Raspberry Liver Pate *(see Page 142 for recipe)* or just enjoy by themselves. They get quite addictive!

INGREDIENTS
- 1/2 cup *(72 g)* arrowroot flour
- Pinch of salt
- 1 teaspoon *(3 g)* garlic powder
- 2 teaspoons *(2 g)* Italian seasoning
- 2 Tablespoons *(30 ml)* avocado oil
- 2-3 Tablespoons *(30-45 ml)* room temperature water

INSTRUCTIONS
1. Preheat oven to 450 F *(230 C)*.
2. Mix all the ingredients well to form a dough *(add 2 Tablespoons of water in initially and add extra water if necessary to form the dough)*. Roll flat and cut into small crackers.
3. Bake for 10-12 minutes. Let cool and enjoy.

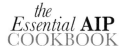

Tropical Trail Mix

Prep Time: 5 minutes
Cook Time: 0 minute
Total Time: 5 minutes
Yield: 1 serving
Serving Size: 1 bowl

Most trail mixes you buy contain lots of non-AIP ingredients like nuts, seeds, seed oils, and sometimes even non-AIP spices. So get some AIP ingredients and make your own for a really quick and easy snack. If you have a dehydrator, then you can also dehydrate all sorts of fruits and vegetables and mix them together to make even more unique AIP trail mixes.

INGREDIENTS

- Equal amounts of freeze-dried berries *(I used raspberry)*, coconut flakes, dried mango slices *(or dried pineapple chunks)*, cut into small pieces

INSTRUCTIONS

1. Combine together.

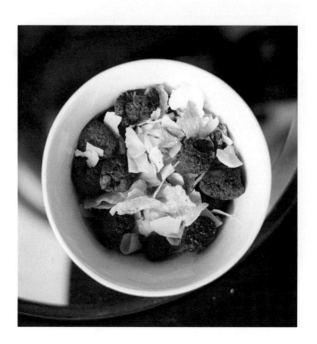

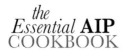

Chapter 7:

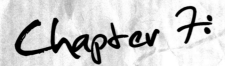

Beverages

Avocado Green Smoothie

Prep Time: 5 minutes
Cook Time: 0 minutes
Total Time: 5 minutes
Yield: 1 serving
Serving Size: 1 glass

INGREDIENTS

- 1/2 ripe avocado
- 1 ripe banana
- 1/2 cup *(120 ml)* coconut water
- 1 handful of greens of your choice *(spinach, kale, chard)*
- 1 cup *(250 g)* ice

INSTRUCTIONS

1. Place all the ingredients into the blender and blend well. Add extra coconut water to help with the blending if necessary.

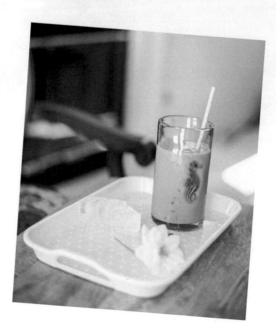

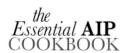

Bone Broth

Prep Time: 5 minutes
Cook Time: 10 hours
Total Time: 10 hours 5 minutes
Yield: 8-16 servings *(depends on size of slow cooker)*
Serving Size: 1 cup *(approx.)*

INGREDIENTS

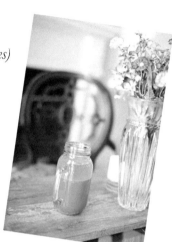

- 3-4 lbs *(1361-1814 g)* of bones *(I typically use beef bones)*
- 1 gallon *(3.8 l)* water *(adjust for your slow cooker size)*
- 2 Tablespoons *(30 ml)* apple cider vinegar
- 1 onion, peeled and chopped
- 1 carrot, peeled and chopped
- 2 Tablespoons *(7.5 g)* parsley
- Salt *(to taste)*

INSTRUCTIONS

1. Add everything to the slow cooker.
2. Cook on the low setting in slow cooker for 10 hours.
3. Cool the broth, then strain and pour broth into a container.
4. Store the broth in the refrigerator until you're ready to use.
5. Scoop out the congealed fat on top of the broth *(optional, but the broth is otherwise very fatty)*.
6. Heat broth when needed.

SUGGESTIONS

• After you've made the first batch of broth, you can make additional batches with the same bones. Typically, bones will last for 4-5 batches of broth.

SUBSTITUTIONS

• Lemon or lime juice *(or anything else acidic)* can be used instead of apple cider vinegar - you can also omit it *(it's often suggested to help draw more minerals out of the bones)*.
• Place a whole chicken into the slow cooker instead of the bones to make chicken broth instead. Shred the chicken meat and use in dishes like Chicken and "Rice" or the Sweet Potato Breakfast Hash.

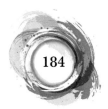

Coconut Iced Tea Latte

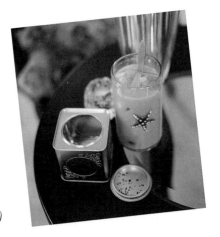

Prep Time: 10 minutes
Cook Time: 0 minutes
Total Time: 10 minutes
Yield: 2 servings
Serving Size: 1 cup

INGREDIENTS

- 2 cups *(480 ml)* black tea
- 3 Tablespoons *(45 ml)* coconut milk *(or to taste)*
- 1 Tablespoon *(15 ml)* honey *(or to taste)*
- Glass of ice *(to serve in)*

INSTRUCTIONS

1. Brew the black tea until ready.
2. Add in the coconut milk and honey to taste. Blend for a few seconds or use a milk frother and pour into a glass with ice.

Cucumber Basil Ice Cubes

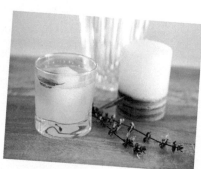

Prep Time: 15 minutes
Cook Time: 0 minutes
Total Time: 15 minutes + 4 hours freezing time
Yield: 2-3 serving
Serving Size: 1 large ice cube

INGREDIENTS

- 1 cucumber *(12 oz or 340 g)*, peeled and cut into large chunks
- 5 small basil leaves
- Juice from 1/4 lime
- 1/4 cup *(60 ml)* water

INSTRUCTIONS

1. Place everything into the blender and blend well. *(If using a juicer, omit the water and add the lime juice in after juicing the cucumber and basil).*
2. Strain the puree and pour the resulting liquid into large ice cube trays or molds.
3. Save the resulting cucumber solids to make the Cold Cucumber Mash *(see Page 134 for recipe).*
4. Freeze the trays for 4-5 hours *(or overnight)* until solid.
5. Make drinks using the ice cubes e.g., add them to sparkling water.

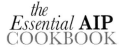

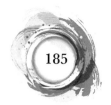

Ginger Basil Tea

Prep Time: 5 minutes
Cook Time: 0 minutes
Total Time: 5 minutes
Yield: 2 servings
Serving Size: 1 cup of tea

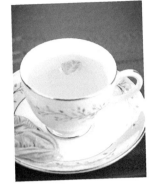

INGREDIENTS

- 2 cups *(480 ml)* boiling water
- 1/2 teaspoon *(0.85 g)* fresh ginger, grated *(or 10 very thin slices of ginger)*
- 4 fresh basil leaves

INSTRUCTIONS

1. Add the ginger and basil to a cup or teapot and pour boiling water into the cup/teapot.
2. Brew for 5 minutes.
3. Press the basil leaves gently with a spoon to get more flavor out of them, if desired.
4. Sieve out *(using a special teapot or a strainer)* the ginger and basil. Enjoy hot or cold.

Hot "Chocolate"

Prep Time: 0 minutes
Cook Time: 10 minutes
Total Time: 10 minutes
Yield: 1 serving
Serving Size: 1 cup

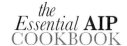

INGREDIENTS

- 1 Tablespoon *(5 g)* carob powder
- 2 teaspoons *(42 g)* raw honey *(or to taste)*
- 1 cup *(240 ml)* coconut milk

INSTRUCTIONS

1. Heat the coconut milk in a saucepan. Add in the carob and raw honey. Mix well and serve hot.

Lemon, Ginger, Honey Tea

Prep Time: 5 minutes
Cook Time: 0 minutes
Total Time: 5 minutes
Yield: 1 serving
Serving Size: 1 cup

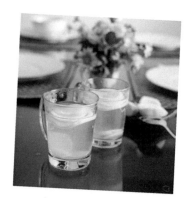

INGREDIENTS

- 1 cup *(240 ml)* boiling water
- 1/2 lemon, cut 3 slices and then squeeze the rest of the juice into the cup
- 3 thin slices of ginger
- Honey *(to taste)*

INSTRUCTIONS

1. Place all the ingredients into a cup.
2. Steep for 5 minutes.

Lemon Thyme Infused Iced Tea

Prep Time: 10 minutes
Cook Time: 0 minutes
Total Time: 10 minutes + overnight infusion
Yield: 6-8 servings
Serving Size: 1 cup

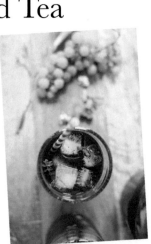

INGREDIENTS

- 4-6 cups *(1-1.5 l)* of black tea
- 6 sprigs of lemon thyme

INSTRUCTIONS

1. Brew the black tea until ready.
2. Remove the tea bag(s) and add 2 sprigs of lemon thyme into the hot tea.
3. Let cool and then refrigerate overnight.
4. Remove the old lemon thyme sprigs and serve with ice and fresh sprigs of lemon thyme for decoration.

SUBSTITUTIONS

- Juice from 1/2 lemon and sprigs of thyme can be used instead of lemon thyme.

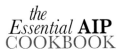

Pomegranate Apple Ginger Fizz

Prep Time: 5 minutes
Cook Time: 0 minutes
Total Time: 5 minutes
Yield: 1 serving
Serving Size: 1 glass

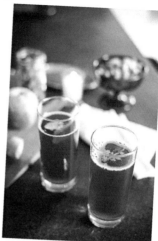

INGREDIENTS

- 1/3 cup *(80 ml)* pomegranate juice
- 2 thin slices of ginger
- 1 cup *(240 ml)* soda water
- 1/2 Tablespoon *(7.5 ml)* apple cider vinegar

INSTRUCTIONS

1. Pour the pomegranate juice and apple cider vinegar into a glass with 2 thin slices of ginger. Top with 1 cup of soda water.

Strawberry Banana Smoothie

Prep Time: 5 minutes
Cook Time: 0 minutes
Total Time: 5 minutes
Yield: 1 serving
Serving Size: 1 glass

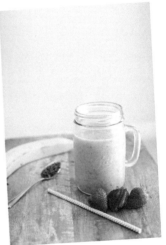

INGREDIENTS

- 8 strawberries
- 1 banana
- 1/2 Tablespoon *(7.5 ml)* coconut oil
- 1/2 cup *(120 ml)* coconut milk
- 1 cup *(250 g)* ice
- 1 teaspoon *(1 g)* mint tea leaves
- Raw honey *(or other sweetener to taste) (optional)*

INSTRUCTIONS

1. Place all the ingredients into the blender and blend well.

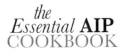

Zingy Salted Lime Soda

Prep Time: 5 minutes
Cook Time: 0 minutes
Total Time: 5 minutes
Yield: 1 serving
Serving Size: 1 glass

INGREDIENTS

- 1 lime, juiced
- 1 and 1/4 cups *(300 ml)* chilled seltzer water *(amount can be adjusted to taste)*
- 1/8 to 1/4 teaspoon *(0.6-1.25 g)* salt *(or to taste)*

INSTRUCTIONS

1. Juice 1 lime and add the chilled seltzer water and salt to the lime juice.
2. Stir gently to dissolve the salt.
3. Serve chilled.

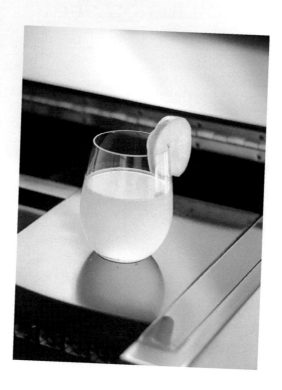

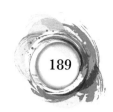

Appendix A: Detailed AIP Food List

FOODS TO EAT ON AIP

VEGETABLES

Pretty much all vegetables except nightshades are good on AIP. Just remember that grains like corn, wheat, and rice are NOT vegetables.

Acorn Squash
Artichoke Hearts
Artichokes
Arugula (Rocket)
Asparagus
Avocado
Beet Top
Beets
Bok Choy
Broccoli
Brussels Sprouts
Butternut Squash
Cabbage
Carrots
Cassava
Cauliflower
Celery
Chinese Cabbage
Chicory
Collard Greens
Cucumber
Dandelion
Endive
Fennel
Fiddleheads
Green Onions

Jerusalem Artichokes
Jicama
Kale
Kohlrabi
Leeks
Lettuce
Mushrooms (All Kinds)
Mustard Greens
Okra
Onions
Parsley
Parsnips
Pumpkin
Radicchio
Radish
Rapini
Romaine Lettuce
Rutabaga
Seaweed (All Sea Vegetables, but avoiding Algae (including chlorella and spirulina)*)
Spaghetti Squash
Spinach
Squash
Sweet Potato

Swiss Chard
Taro
Turnips
Turnip Greens
Watercress
Yellow Crookneck Squash
Yellow Squash
Yam
Zucchini

LEGUMES

Almost all legumes are off limits, but green beans and peas are actually still in seed form and fine to eat generally (Sarah Ballantyne states to avoid them initially).

* indicates that the food is not allowed on Sarah Ballantyne's version of AIP.

the **AIP**
Essential
COOKBOOK

FRUITS
(Limit to 2-5 portions per day for Sarah Ballantyne's version)

Most fruits are different than they were a million years ago, but some are healthier than others. Here are the best:

Blackberry
Blueberry
Coconut
Cranberry
Raspberry
Olive
Avocado

Here are some other fruits to consider:

Apples
Apricot

Bananas
Cantaloupe
Cherries
Dates
Figs
Grapefruit
Grapes
Guava
Honeydew Melon
Kiwi
Lemon
Lime
Lychee
Mango
Nectarines
Oranges
Papaya
Passion Fruit

Peaches
Pears
Persimmon
Pineapple
Plums
Pomegranates
Rhubarb
Star Fruit
Strawberry
Tangerine
Watermelon

NOTE: Cape Gooseberries, Garden Huckleberries, and Goji Berries are Nightshades and are on the Not Allowed Food List for AIP.

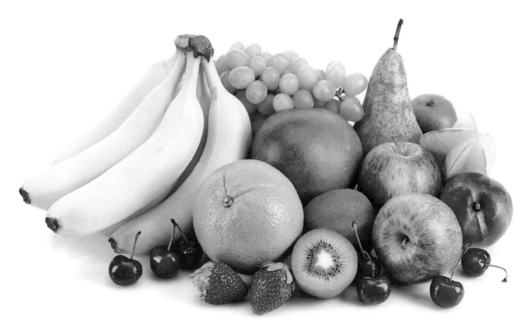

MEATS

Every meat is good, but quality makes a difference. Buy grass-fed, wild, and pastured when applicable and possible.
Check out US Wellness Meats if you want high quality meat delivered to your door - http://paleomagazine.com/us-wellness-meats

Alligator
Bear
Beef
Bison
Chicken
Deer
Duck
Elk
Goat
Goose
Kangaroo
Lamb
Moose
Pheasant
Pork

Quail
Rabbit
Reindeer
Sheep
Snake
Turkey
Veal
Wild Boar
Wild Turkey

ORGAN MEATS /OFFAL
There is no other category of food that is as nutritious as organ meats. Eat any of the

following from pretty much any animal:
Heart
Liver
Kidney
Bone Marrow
Tongue
Tripe
Blood
Skin
Rinds
Brain
Sweetbreads
Tail

FISH AND SEAFOOD

Fish is highly nutritious, but buy wild-caught fish whenever possible. And, apart from organ meats, shellfish is pretty much the most nutrient-dense food you can eat.

Anchovies
Bass
Cod
Eel
Haddock
Halibut
Mackerel
Mahi Mahi
Orange Roughy
Perch

Red Snapper
Rockfish
Salmon
Sardines
Tilapia
Tuna
Sole
Grouper
Turbot
Trout

Shark
Abalone
Clams
Crab
Lobster
Mussels
Oysters
Shrimp
Scallops

Appendix A: Detailed AIP Food List

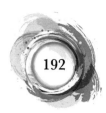

FOODS TO EAT ON AIP

COOKING OILS

Pay particular attention to the oils that you cook in. These can make a huge difference in your overall health.

Avocado Oil

Coconut Oil

Lard

Tallow

Olive Oil

Palm Oil (but not palm kernel oil)

Duck Fat

Truffle Oil

Red Palm Oil

Bacon Fat

Leaf Lard

Pan Drippings

Salo

Schmaltz

Strutto

HERBS AND SPICES

Lemon balm

Basil Leaves

Bay Leaves

Chamomile

Chervil

Chives

Cilantro

Cinnamon

Cloves

Dill Weed

Garlic

Ginger

Horseradish

Lavender

Mace

Marjoram

Onion powder/flakes

Oregano

Parsley

Peppermint

Rosemary

Saffron

Sage

Salt

Savory

Spearmint

Tarragon

Thyme

Turmeric (requires some caution)

Lemongrass

Lime Leaves

Wasabi

FRUITS AND BERRIES THAT ARE USED AS SPICES

(Sarah Ballantyne recommends eliminating these initially)

Allspice

Star Anise

Caraway

Cardamom

Juniper

Black Pepper

White Pepper

Green Peppercorn

Pink Peppercorn

Vanilla Bean (including vanilla extract - might be ok if cooked)

Sumac

Appendix A: Detailed AIP Food List

FOODS TO EAT ON AIP

FERMENTED AND OTHER FOODS

Pay particular attention to the oils that you cook in. These can make a huge difference in your overall health.

FERMENTED FOODS

Note - check any pre-made foods for non-AIP ingredients)

Water kefir
Coconut kefir
Coconut yogurt
Fermented sauerkraut
Kombucha
(make sure you buy or make ones with live cultures and without additives or extra sugar, and if following Sarah Ballantyne's version, to buy ones without thickeners)

OTHER FOODS

Anchovies
Cocoa (or 100% chocolate) (not permitted on Sarah Ballantyne's version)
Coffee (not permitted on Sarah Ballantyne's version)
Tea (herbal, green, black)
Gluten-Free Alcohol (not permitted for drinking on Sarah Ballantyne's version - ok to use in cooking if it's cooked off)
Vinegars (including apple cider, coconut water vinegar, red wine, white wine, balsamic)
Coconut aminos
Fish Sauce
Capers

Organic Jams and Chutneys
Gelatin
Coconut Water
Coconut Milk Kefir
Coconut Milk (no emulsifiers)
Beet and Other Vegetable Kvass
Kombucha
Green Juices
Agar Agar
Arrowroot Powder
Baking Soda
Carob Powder
Coconut Butter
Coconut Cream
Green Banana Flour
Cream of Tartar
Kuzu Starch
Plantain Flour
Water Chestnut Flour
Tiger Nut

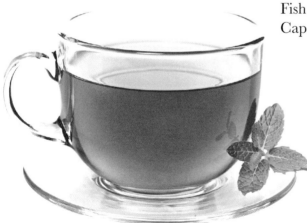

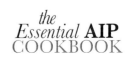

Appendix A: Detailed AIP Food List

the **Essential AIP** COOKBOOK

FOODS NOT ALLOWED ON AIP

SWEETENERS, VEGETABLE AND SEED OILS

Sugar
Honey**
Coconut Sugar
High Fructose Corn
Syrup
Maple Syrup**
Artificial Sweeteners
Agave
Maltodextrin
Corn Syrup
Molasses**
Pomegranate Molasses**
Date Sugar**

Rice Syrup
Any Soda
Any Candy
Stevia
Coconut Sugar

Corn oil
Canola oil
Vegetable oil
Soybean oil
Shortening
Sunflower oil
Safflower oil
Cottonseed oil
Grapeseed oil
Peanut oil
Margarine
Palm kernel oil
Nut oils

GRAINS, NUTS, AND SEEDS

Wheat
Barley
Corn
Millet
Oats
Rice
Rye
Sorghum
Spelt
Pasta
Bread
Crackers
Cookies
Waffles
Pancakes
Pizza
Rice Cakes
Quinoa (even though it's
not technically a grain)

Almonds
Brazil Nuts
Hazelnuts
Macadamias
Pecans
Pine Nuts
Pistachios
Pumpkin Seeds
Sesame Seeds
Sunflower Seeds
Walnuts
Chestnuts

SPICES THAT ARE SEEDS

Anise Seed
Annatto Seed
Black Caraway
Celery Seed
Coriander Seed
Cumin
Dill Seed
Fennel Seed
Fenugreek
Mustard Seed
Nutmeg
Poppy Seed
Sesame Seed

**May be allowed in moderation under Sarah Ballantyne's version.

Appendix A: Detailed AIP Food List

FOODS NOT ALLOWED ON AIP

DAIRY, LEGUMES, AND NIGHTSHADES

DAIRY
Milk
Ice Cream
Frozen Yogurt
Yogurt
Cream
Sour Cream
Dairy Kefir
Ghee
Butter

LEGUMES
Garbanzo Beans
Black Beans
Kidney Beans
Mung Beans
Lima Beans
Chickpeas
Black-Eyed Peas
Lentils
Snow Peas

Sugar Snap Peas
Peanuts
Soybeans
Tofu
Soymilk
White Beans
Pinto Beans
Fava Beans
Red Beans

NIGHTSHADES
Ashwagandha
Capsicums
Potatoes
Tomatoes
Tomatillos
Peppers (of any kind)
Cocona
Garden Huckleberries
Kutjera
Naranjillas

Pepinos
Pimentos
Tamarillos
Eggplants/aubergines
Goji berries
Cape Gooseberries
Cayenne pepper
Paprika spice
Chili powder
Red Pepper Flakes
Chili Pepper Flakes
Curry spice powder
Garam Masala spice
Most spice blends
Paleo ketchup
Curry Powder
Red Pepper
Chinese Five-Spice
Powder
Steak Seasoning

Additional Resources

BOOKS
The Paleo Approach by Sarah Ballantyne
The Autoimmune Solution by Amy Myers
The Wahls Protocol by Terry Wahls
The Root Cause by Izabella Wentz

**WEBSITES ON PALEO/
AUTOIMMUNE SCIENCE**
www.chriskresser.com
www.thepaleomom.com
www.perfecthealthdiet.com
www.drknews.com

WEBSITES WITH AIP RECIPES
www.paleomagazine.com/autoimmune-paleo-recipes
www.thepaleomom.com
www.phoenixhelix.com
www.alt-ternativeautoimmune.com
www.nutrisclerosis.com
www.acleanplate.com
www.healingfamilyeats.com
www.thebaconmum.com

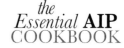

the **AIP**
Essential
COOKBOOK

Appendix C:
4-Week AIP Meal Plan

ABOUT THIS MEAL PLAN

This is a 4-week meal plan using recipes from this cookbook.

This meal plan is *designed for 2 people* and covers breakfast, lunch, and dinner.

Important note: 1 batch means to make the recipe as stated, 2 batches means to make a double portion of the recipe.

Week 1

Day 1:
Breakfast: Make 2 batches of Blueberry Mint Smoothie (page 22).
Lunch: Make 1 batch of Orange Beef Stir-Fry (page 88).
Dinner: Make 2 batches of Beets "No-Tomato" Chili (page 79) with 1 batch of Baked Spaghetti Squash (page 132) (or grated zucchini or cucumber if you don't have spaghetti squash available). Refrigerate 1 batch of the beets chili.

Day 2:
Breakfast: Make 1 batch of Apple Cauliflower Porridge (page 20).
Lunch: Make 1 batch of Mango and Chicken Salad with Coconut Caesar Dressing (page 64). Cook some extra chicken and refrigerate for future salads this week.
Dinner: Reheat rest of the beets chili from Day 1.

Day 3:
Breakfast: Make 1 batch of Amazing Banana Pancakes (page 18).
Lunch: Make a salad with leftover chicken from Day 2 lunch.
Dinner: Make 2 batches of Grilled Chicken Drumsticks with Garlic Marinade (page 61) with 1 batch of Creamy Mashed Sweet Potatoes (page 136). Refrigerate 1 batch of the drumsticks and sweet potato mash.

Day 4:
Breakfast: Make 1 batch of Carrot and Apple Hash with Cinnamon and Ginger (page 25).
Lunch: Make 1 batch of Fish Tacos with Plum Salsa (page 118).
Dinner: Reheat chicken drumsticks and make 1 batch of Fried Sweet Plantains (page 139).

Day 5:
Breakfast: Make 2 batches of Perfect Green Smoothie (page 34).
Lunch: Make 2 batches of Cucumber Ginger Shrimp (page 116).
Dinner: Make 1 batch of Filet Mignon with Mushroom Sauce (page 84) and enjoy with rest of mashed sweet potatoes from Day 3.

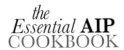

Day 6:
Breakfast: Make 2 batches of Carrot Apple Banana Smoothie (page 26).
Lunch: Make 1 batch of Easy Bacon Brussels Sprouts (page 137). Eat 1/2 batch and refrigerate the rest.
Dinner: Make 2 batches of Arrowroot Battered Fish (page 110) with 1/2 batch of Parsnip Fries (page 144).

Day 7:
Breakfast: Make 1 batch of Chicken and Apple Sausages (page 27) and eat 1/2 batch and freeze rest.
Lunch: Reheat rest of the Brussels sprouts from Day 6.
Dinner: Make 1 batch of Turmeric Veggie "Curry" (page 128) with 1 batch of Cauliflower White "Rice" (page 133).

Week 2
Day 1:
Breakfast: Reheat premade Chicken and Apple Sausages (1/2 batch) (page 27).
Lunch: Make 1/2 batch of Baked Salmon with Cabbage, Apple, and Fennel (page 112).
Dinner: Make 1 batch of Pressure Cooker Jamaican Oxtail Stew (page 126). Eat 1/2 batch and refrigerate the rest.

Day 2:
Breakfast: Make 1 batch of Chicken, Bacon, and Apple Mini Meatloaves (page 28) and eat 1/2 batch and refrigerate rest.
Lunch: Reheat rest of oxtail stew from Day 1.
Dinner: Make 1 batch of Pan-Fried Pork Tenderloin (page 102) with 2 batches of Garlic Lemon Broccolini Saute (page 140). Refrigerate 1 batch of the broccolini saute.

Day 3:
Breakfast: Reheat premade Chicken, Bacon, and Apple Mini Meatloaves (1/2 batch) (page 28).
Lunch: Make 1 batch of Broccoli Beef (page 80) with 2 batches of Cauliflower White "Rice" (page 133). Eat 1 batch of cauliflower white rice and refrigerate the rest.
Dinner: Make 2 batches of Italian Seasoning Crusted Lamb (page 124) and enjoy with rest of the broccolini saute from Day 2.

Day 4:
Breakfast: Make 2 batches of Perfect Green Smoothie (page 34).
Lunch: Make 1 batch of Steak Medallions with Ginger Asparagus Mushroom Saute (page 86).
Dinner: Make 1/2 batch of "Breaded" Fish with Garlic Sauce (page 115) with 1/2 batch of Parsnip Fries (page 144).

Day 5:
Breakfast: Make 1 batch of Spinach, Mushroom, Bacon Saute (page 35).
Lunch: Make 1 batch of Fish and Leek Saute (page 117) and enjoy with rest of the cauliflower rice from Day 3.
Dinner: Make 1 batch of Bacon Acorn Squash Mash (page 99).
Prep: Make 1 batch of Bone Broth (page 183) in the slow cooker.

Day 6:
Breakfast: Make 1 batch of Bone Broth Noodle Soup (page 24) using premade Bone Broth (page

Appendix C: 4-Week AIP Meal Plan

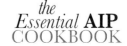

the
Essential **AIP**
COOKBOOK

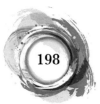

183).
Lunch: Make 2 batches of Blueberry Liver Stir-Fry (page 123).
Dinner: Make 1/2 batch of Chinese Pork Spare Ribs (page 100).

Day 7:
Breakfast: Make 1 batch of "Chocolate" Avocado Smoothie (page 30).
Lunch: Make 1 batch of Rosemary Baked Salmon (page 121) with 1 batch of Creamy Cauliflower Mash (page 135).
Dinner: Make 1 batch of Pressure Cooker Beef Short Ribs (page 92) (eat 1/2 batch and refrigerate rest) with 1/2 batch of Splendid Strawberry Spinach Salad (page 58).
Prep: Make 1 batch of Slow Cooker Shredded Pork (page 108).

Week 3
Day 1:
Breakfast: Make 1 batch of Sweet Potato Breakfast Hash (page 36) using the leftover Pressure Cooker Beef Short Ribs (page 92).
Lunch: Make 1 batch of Pineapple Pork (page 104) using the slow cooker shredded pork.
Dinner: Make 1 batch of Broccoli Beef (page 80) with 2 batches of Cold Cucumber Mash (page 134).

Day 2:
Breakfast: Make 2 batches Perfect Green Smoothie (page 34).
Lunch: Saute rest of the slow cooker pork with some garlic and onions.
Dinner: Make 1 batch of Sweet Potato Guacamole Burger (page 94) with 1/2 batch of Parsnip Fries (page 144).
Prep: Make more bone broth (page 183) if you're out.

Day 3:
Breakfast: Make 1 batch of Amazing Banana Pancakes (page 18).
Lunch: Make 1 batch of Rosemary Baked Salmon (page 121) and enjoy with a salad.
Dinner: Make 1 batch of Vietnamese Beef Pho (page 96) using premade Bone Broth (page 183).

Day 4:
Breakfast: Make 1 batch of "Chocolate" Avocado Smoothie (page 30).
Lunch: Make 2 batches of Easy Tuna Salad (page 48). Save 1 batch for tomorrow.
Dinner: Make 1 batch of Filet Mignon with Mushroom Sauce (page 84) with 1 batch of Apple Bacon Brussels Sprouts (page 131).

Day 5:
Breakfast: Make 1 batch of Amazing Banana Pancakes (page 18).
Lunch: Eat rest of tuna salad from Day 4.
Dinner: Make 1 batch of Chinese Meatball Soup (page 82) with premade Bone Broth (page 183).
Prep: Marinate the Marinated Grilled Flank Steak (1 batch) (page 87).

Day 6:
Breakfast: Make 1 batch of Bone Broth Noodle Soup (page 24) using premade Bone Broth (page 183).
Lunch: Make 1 batch of Thai Chicken Pad See Ew (page 76).
Dinner: Make 1 batch of Marinated Grilled Flank Steak (page 87) with 1 batch of Garlic Lemon Broccolini Saute (page 140). Refrigerate 1/3 batch of steak for tomorrow.

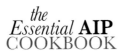

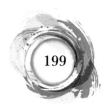

Day 7:
Breakfast: Make 1 batch of Apple Cauliflower Porridge (page 20).
Lunch: Make salad with 1/3 batch of premade flank steak from Day 6.
Dinner: Make 1 batch of Slow Cooker Beef Stew (page 93) (eat 1/3 and refrigerate the rest).
Prep: Set the slow cooker in the morning for the Slow Cooker Beef Stew (page 93).

Week 4

Day 1:
Breakfast: Make 1 batch of Sweet Potato Breakfast Hash (page 36) using 1/3 batch of premade flank steak from Day 6.
Lunch: Make 2 batches of Honey Glazed Chicken Drumsticks (page 62) with 1 batch of Garlic Lemon Broccolini Saute (page 140). Refrigerate 1 batch of chicken drumsticks.
Dinner: Reheat 1/3 batch of beef stew from day before.
Prep: Make more bone broth (page 183) if you're out.

Day 2:
Breakfast: Make 1 batch of Bone Broth Noodle Soup (page 24) using premade Bone Broth (page 183).
Lunch: Make 1/2 batch of Chicken and "Rice" (page 74) using chicken meat from rest of chicken drumsticks from Day 1.
Dinner: Reheat rest of beef stew (1/3 batch) from Day 7.
Prep: Make 1 batch of Slow Cooker Bacon & Chicken (page 72).

Day 3:
Breakfast: Make 1 batch of Carrot and Apple Hash with Cinnamon and Ginger (page 25).
Lunch: Eat 1/3 batch of premade slow cooker bacon & chicken with a simple salad.
Dinner: Make 1 batch of Vietnamese Beef Pho (page 96) with premade Bone Broth (page 183).

Day 4:
Breakfast: Make 1 batch of Spinach, Mushroom, Bacon Saute (page 35).
Lunch: Eat 1/3 batch of premade slow cooker bacon & chicken with a simple salad.
Dinner: Make 1 batch of Steak Medallions with Ginger Asparagus Mushroom Saute (page 86).

Day 5:
Breakfast: Make 2 batches of Blueberry Mint Smoothie (page 22).
Lunch: Make 1 batch of Sweet Potato Guacamole Burger (page 94) with 1 cup each of premade Bone Broth (page 183).
Dinner: Make 1 batch of Pineapple Fried "Rice" (page 68).

Day 6:
Breakfast: Make 1 batch of Apple Cauliflower Porridge (page 20).
Lunch: Make 1 batch of Korean BBQ Beef (page 85). Refrigerate 1/2 batch.
Dinner: Make 1 batch of Mango and Chicken Salad with Coconut Caesar Dressing (page 64).

Day 7:
Breakfast: Make 1 batch of Amazing Banana Pancakes (page 18).
Lunch: Reheat rest of BBQ beef from Day 6 and eat with a simple salad.
Dinner: Saute rest (1/3 batch) of slow cooker bacon & chicken with asparagus and mushrooms.

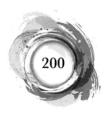

Recipe Index

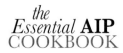

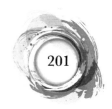

Recipe Index

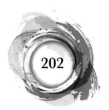

Recipe Index

Fotolia.com (c)- Picture Partners, cachecache, katrinshine, Alena Ozerova, darkbird, airdone, aliaksei_7799, Anterovium, Dionisvera, valery121283, Witold Krasowski, Jiri Hera, Tim UR, Valentina R., sommai, Serhiy Shullye, Africa Studio, Abel Tumik, Mariusz Blach, Cadebou, Grafvision, Nataliia Pyzhova, Popova Olga, volff, mates, Luis Carlos Jiménez, torsakarin, whitestorm, baibaz , goir

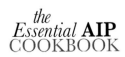
the
Essential **AIP**
COOKBOOK